Patricia McCarthy Faust, MGS

The Boomer Brain

*For Baby Boomers Concerned
About Dementia and Alzheimer's*

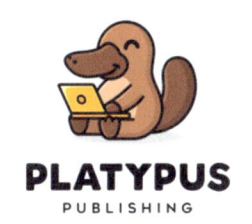

PLATYPUS
PUBLISHING

First published by Platypus Publishing 2024

Copyright © 2024 by Patricia McCarthy Faust, MGS

All rights reserved. No part of this publication may be reproduced, stored or transmitted in any form or by any means, electronic, mechanical, photocopying, recording, scanning, or otherwise without written permission from the publisher. It is illegal to copy this book, post it to a website, or distribute it by any other means without permission.

First edition

ISBN: 978-1-962133-61-6

Dedication

The term 'it takes a village' is not more appropriate than in the writing of this book. I would like to dedicate this to family, mentors, and friends I have been blessed to welcome into my life. It is their encouragement that has driven me to learn how we can all prevent Alzheimer's in our lifetime.

foreword

It's my distinct pleasure to be asked to write a foreword for Patricia Faust's book "The Boomer Brain".

I've had wonderful conversations on this topic with her. There is always something new and topical that Pat brings to the table. The Boomer Brain is evidence of this. Over the past few years as brain health has become important for aging seniors, I've had the honor of having her present on this topic to members at Fitness Over 50 here in Corvallis Oregon.

Patricia is a student of this topic and is always learning more, and improving her content in this area. The Boomer Brain captures her knowledge in a digestible way. This book is a must-read for all ages but is a critical how-to guide for those of us in our sixties, seventies, and older.

Mike Waters MA
Director of Health Promotion
Fitness Over 50
Corvallis Oregon

preface

In 2004 I graduated from Miami University with a master's degree in Gerontology. I was also 53 years old. My excitement to share my knowledge was palpable. My experience was disheartening. I couldn't find my footing as a way forward.

Along came the annual American Society of Aging conference, where I was first introduced to brain health. It was transformative for me. I felt like I found the fountain of youth. We could change our brains! Over the next few years, I found teachers, read research articles, and accumulated certifications. Finally, it was time to spread the word.

What I didn't expect was that it was still too early for people to listen to me. I was met with indifference. For a few years, I worked with Dr. Paul Nussbaum as his corporate wellness director. Dr. Nussbaum was one of the first experts to explain the benefits of brain health and brain function. I thought it would be an easy process to get companies to understand how brain health could benefit their wellness programming. At that time wellness initiatives encompassed everything from the neck down. They couldn't comprehend that the brain was running everything. But I couldn't sell it. I presented before a group of retired executives to gain some insights on how to proceed. They were emphatic in their belief that this was a valuable program. But (the dreaded -but), corporations weren't ready for brain health, on how to proceed. They predicted that I would spend at least ten years educating executives about the benefits of brain-healthy employees, and then someone would come in and close the sale. And that is exactly the way it happened!

The science of brain aging, and brain health was just starting to gain some traction when the leading-edge Boomers were in their forties and fifties. The science was just starting to show that with a healthy lifestyle, we could change our brains. There wasn't any definitive research to support that we could prevent Alzheimer's just yet. We were uncomfortable with the aging losses we experienced, but we used denial as a coping mechanism even though we were secretly terrified when we couldn't find our car in a parking lot. There was more fear over a diagnosis of Alzheimer's than cancer.

The truth is, we can still change our brains in our sixties, seventies, and beyond. We have the power to delay or even prevent Alzheimer's disease. But we need to know what we must do to make change happen. We all deserve a chance to sidestep Alzheimer's by knowing what to do. We all deserve to have a healthy brain no matter what our age is.

And that is why I wrote this book.

acknowledgements

There is one person who deserves my sincere thanks for completing this book. For years my husband Russ kept nudging me to write a book. And even though I didn't act on it immediately, he kept me thinking about it. When I finally decided that I could do this, Russ became my sounding board, reader, interior book designer, and creative director. His encouragement throughout the writing process was instrumental in getting this book done. I want to thank you Russ for helping me make this happen.

My sons, Russ and Tim, and daughter-in-law, Amy, cheered me through the experience. It was uplifting to know they were behind me sending good energy my way. My two oldest granddaughters, Greer, and Ellah were so enthusiastic about my efforts, and it felt special to have them look up to me. Thank you, family, for your unending support.

A special thanks needs to go out to a couple of friends who really came through for me.

Debbie Hampton, founder of The Best Brain Possible, has written three books. Her knowledge about the brain is extensive. Debbie was one of my readers and her experience was invaluable in making my book better. Thank you, Debbie, for helping me write the best version of my book.

Judy Aufdemkampe is a good friend from our younger days. Judy was an editor years ago and she graciously accepted the challenge of editing my book. Thank you, Judy, for your detailed editing. I am grateful.

Finally, I want to thank my mom. Mom was my biggest cheerleader. She came to hear me speak, lobbied for me to conduct a 5-week course on Memory at the Senior Center where she was a member, and always told me to write a book! She was persistent in that request. Since I hadn't acted on writing this book, her request became an order. So, I promised her I would get it done. Unfortunately, she died before I started writing but my promise to her was continually top-of-mind. It is with great satisfaction that now I can say, "Promise Kept!"

endorsements

The information in The Boomer Brain will help put your brain at ease. Not because the statistics regarding brain decline and projections for Alzheimer's she provides aren't shocking enough, but because this book tells us, in plain English, exactly what we can do on a daily basis to build a healthier brain at any age and lower our risk of decline with age. Pat shares her personal story, insights, and the science behind building a better brain in a way that is interesting, understandable, and doable. Read this book. Your brain will thank you.

Debbie Hampton/The Best Brain Possible

"Chock-full of innovative and actionable advice, The Boomer Brain is a paradigm-shifting, hope-fueled manual that dispels the long-held belief that we are at the mercy of aging. Patricia Faust empowers readers to transform the way they care for their brain and take back the beauty of their life."

Erin Matlock/Founder of Brain Summit

"Pat has written a comprehensive guide to understanding and navigating the intricacies of cognitive ageing, 'The Boomer Brain' is a beacon of hope for those seeking to enrich their later years."

Dr. Sarah McKay/Founder of The Neuroscience Academy

Thank you kindly to Patricia Faust for creating for us a 'Longevity Guide'. Her writing is nourishment for the near retirement and absolute instructive fuel for thought and Self-Action in any realm of aging actively. Faust assertively encourages us to be aware of self-advocacy as a way of better living to our fullest. Her determination and commitment to do the WORK to make a change in aging is inspiring and motivational to each of us who desires to maintain and renew.

Adrienne Walker Hoard, MFA, EdD/Creator/Artivist

"Through Patricia Faust's journey of career change and lived experience, this book delivers a powerful message: brain health is within reach for everyone. Blending together scientific insights and relatable anecdotes, Pat empowers readers to embark on their own journey toward a healthier brain. A read that can motivate all of us to take proactive steps in nurturing the health of our brain."

Dr. Krystal L. Culler, DBH, MA/Founder of the Virtual Brain Health Center

contents

Foreward ii

Preface iii

Acknowledements v

Endorsements vii

Chapter 1 1

Chapter 2 7

Chapter 3 15

Chapter 4 25

Chapter 5 33

Chapter 6 43

Chapter 7 53

Chapter 8 65

Chapter 9 139

Chapter 10 151

Sources 158

Conclusion 161

About the Author 165

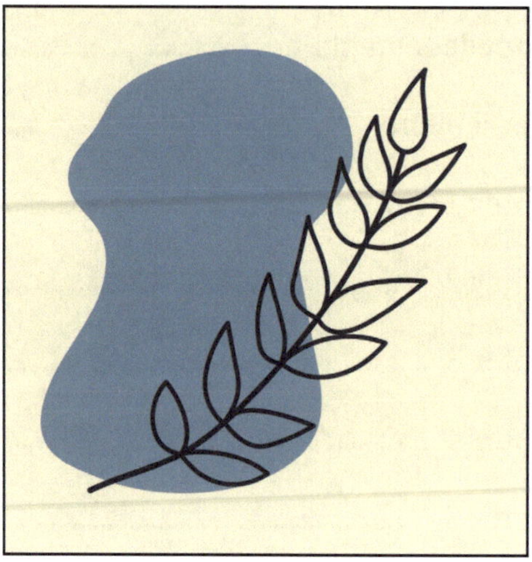

chapter one

Beginnings

During the 1990s I made a complete career shift. I pivoted from being a medical lab technologist to working in nursing homes with occupational and physical therapists. It was a mid-life transition. At that time, I was seeing nursing home residents who had dementia. Back then these units weren't called "Memory Care" but rather "lock-down" units. There was a nun overseeing one of these units in Springfield, Ohio, who took the time to explain to me what being "demented" was about. She flat out said that I was probably thinking that a demented person was the crazy lady locked in the attic! And unfortunately, that was the picture in my head. At that time those with behavior problems due to having dementia were typically given an anti-psychotic drug and seated in front of a TV. I was distraught when I saw that, and it motivated me to change my life.

During the next five years, I embarked on an educational marathon that included getting a BA in Gerontology, a Nursing Home Administrator's license, and finally a Master's in Gerontological Studies. Even though I was in my fifties when I finished these degrees, I was still younger than the people I was working with, and everything I saw and learned was from observing them. I didn't have any family who had dementia, but the older I got the more I feared the small signs that my brain was not as sharp as it used to be. Was I getting dementia?

There was very little written or published about the aging brain at that time. It was widely accepted that the brain we had by our mid-twenties was the best it would be and would start to decline until we died. There was nothing we could do about that. When I saw the devastation of dementia and then started experiencing my own brain aging changes – I was terrified.

Then by chance, I attended a Conference on Aging, and I looked across the exhibition hall and saw a booth about Brain Fitness. What I learned that day – rocked my world! I still had control and I could change my brain! The years that followed were filled with learning all the nuances of the aging brain and how to prevent dementia. I knew that if I was worried about getting Alzheimer's disease, many more people my age were probably worried too.

What I did determine at that time were common boomer brain fears.
- Lost words
- Forgotten names
- Memory lapses
- Slow thinking
- Dementia!!

There were also denials. Maybe I was a little over-enthusiastic when I learned about the capabilities of changing our brains. My thinking was that everyone would want to know how to take care of their brain and prevent Alzheimer's. What I discovered was very unsettling to me.

My excitement peaked around 2008-2009. For the past few years, I have done a deep dive into learning about our brain's aging losses, and how we can recover these losses. We can prevent Alzheimer's Disease (although I couldn't make that claim back then). Instead of reciprocal excitement, I received lots of denial-

- "I am too old to change."
- "It is already too late for me."
- "My mom had Alzheimer's; I probably am going to get it too."

And then there were the fellow boomers who just blew me off. It felt like my words were getting lost in the wind. My final impression was that people were fearful of getting Alzheimer's disease. Denial offered a type of respite from the truth. Unfortunately, denial does not delay or prevent Alzheimer's disease.

We must look at the reality that we are getting older. The one non-modifiable risk factor for getting dementia that works against us as we get older is age. After age 65, the risk doubles every 5 years. According to the Alzheimer's Association 2023 Facts and Figures, the prevalence of people 85+ living with Alzheimer's disease is 2.37 million (35.4%). There is no denial, or excuse that can change this statistic.

There is also the wear and tear on the brain the longer we live.

We don't live in a bubble, and we must always be adapting to our environment. Our environment can be joyful with family and friends and purpose; or it can be challenging filled with hardship due to illness, loss, or sedentary lifestyle choices. The lessons we learn and take with us can help us navigate life's choppy waters. Or, we can succumb to toxic stress and have a future filled with difficulty. All of us probably have tales to tell, but I want to drive home the point that it is never too late to change your brain!

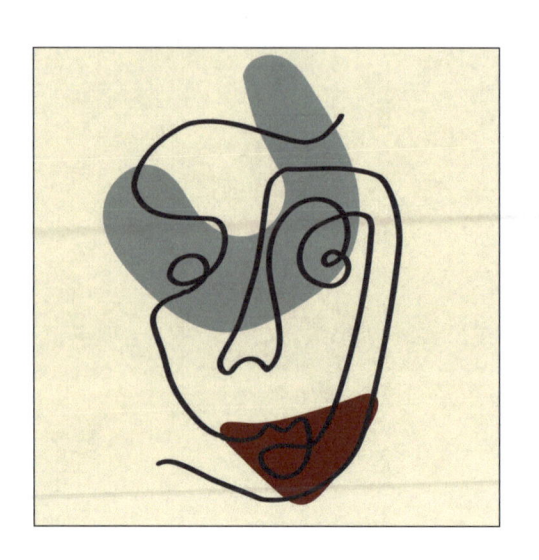

chapter two

Brain Aging Changes Can Be Terrifying!

Thinking back to my 'younger' years is both scary and comforting. As an overachiever, I consistently met the goals that I had set for myself. My brain was my best friend. The three-pound organ between my ears never let me down. Throughout my forties I made big changes in my life. In that decade I began working in a hospital clinical laboratory. This was my dream job and my first real job at that time. The daily challenges of medical science lit up my brain. But what excited me the most, eventually bored me. Once the challenge of new learning was gone, the job became very repetitive, making me feel like a production line worker. This would turn out to be a pattern for me; once the challenge was over, boredom takes over. Initially, I changed the lab setting. After the hospital, I went to an industrial complex and supervised the lab in the medical department. This was as far away from a hospital setting as I could get. The challenge for my brain was not doing the lab work, but rather functioning in a setting where everything was not sterile. It was quite an adjustment.

Having conquered that, I yearned for another change.

It was time to go back to a professional medical environment, where I felt like I was contributing to people's health. I was fortunate to find a job at a lab that did the lab work for eight dialysis clinics in three states. This job enabled me to work on some research studies, and perform lab testing on dialysis patients who were medically challenging. This was my new dream job and I believe I would have stayed there but the powers to be decided to close our site.

In a series of outside the lab jobs over the next ten years, I learned to begin to teach myself whatever I needed to know. My brain was in overdrive as I navigated through this chaotic time. The transitions were scary because I was starting all over in careers that were totally new to me. Of course, my brain loved the change, and I excelled. But, just as before, my brain became bored with the day-to-day routine. Once the challenge was gone, I got restless, and searched for a new job to feel the energy of accomplishment again. The last career of that era was medical sales. I became quite good at that. Financially, I did well in sales and even though I was bored, I probably would not have left the security of that income.

Trying to Make My Brain Function Faster
But the universe had other plans for me, and in November 1997 I had two automobile accidents in three weeks. They were both serious accidents and I sustained injuries that would be with me forever. Those injuries took me out of sales because I couldn't spend all day on the road going from client to client. It was time to decide what I was going to do for the rest of my working life. I went on a five-year learning marathon. In one week, I registered at the Ohio

Academy of Holistic Health to receive certification in Clinical Aromatherapy. That same week I registered at the Mount St. Joseph University in Cincinnati to receive a BA in Gerontology and acquired a Nursing Home Administrators license. This period of my life alerted me to the fact that my brain just wasn't as sharp as it used to be. Working exceptionally hard to keep up with assignments, critical thinking as an older student made me doubt myself. Even though I didn't realize it at the time, I was giving my brain, and therefore myself, the best gift ever. After a short period of time my academic workload became more fluid and easier. I was thinking faster and able to keep up with the younger students. I actually felt younger!

The last two years of this learning marathon were spent at Miami University in Oxford, Ohio. I accepted an assistantship to attend Graduate School to obtain a master's degree in Gerontological Studies. This was an unplanned goal I thought was out of my reach but there I was – in grad school! If I was surprised at my slow brain function in undergraduate school, I was overwhelmed at how deficient I felt trying to keep up with my classmates. Now at this point they were 25 and I was 50 years old. They were wicked smart. For the first few weeks I came home and cried, did homework, and went to bed. I felt like a deer in headlights; what had I done to myself? But again, by pushing my brain to function at a higher level I was challenging my brain to accomplish more than I imagined possible! Those couple of years in grad school changed my brain and my life. I felt younger physically and mentally. It wasn't until later when I learned about my aging brain and how I could change it. I had created a brain years younger than my chronological age!

A Life-Changing Brain Event
That was the perfect scenario for brain aging, but the following years would be more difficult. After years of balance dysfunction from Meniere's disease, I had brain surgery in 2012 and I was not prepared for the length of my recovery. My challenges were to retrain my brain so that the left side of my brain would take over complete balance function for the right side of my brain. At this point I was familiar with the power of neurogenesis (growing new neurons) and neuroplasticity (the ability to change form and function). This was a huge task for my brain to accomplish and it didn't happen quickly. Through balance rehab therapy I learned the proper exercises to start creating the new neural pathways for the left side of my brain to be the total balance master. What I didn't expect, and no one told me – it would take three years of continual balance exercises for me to reach the point where I wasn't so horribly dizzy, and I could walk a straight line. But I DID IT! It was a hard-earned miracle.

My other challenge from the surgery was to get my high-functioning brain back. I was under anesthesia for five hours. My brain was inflamed from the surgery itself. I could barely think for a few weeks. By then I started becoming frustrated because recovery was so hard. Since I had extensive knowledge of brain health and function, I did ten-minutes of brain exercises each morning targeting speed of processing, focus, concentration, memory. By targeting specific functions, I was able to move my brain through the brain fog I was experiencing. This, too, took time. The brain makes changes through repetition and consistency. I had to keep doing these exercises every day until I felt my brain function and capacity start to feel normal again, and normal became a reality.

These were life-changing brain events for me. Going back to grad school brought the cognitive aging losses front and center for me to see. When you are with people who are the same age as you, you don't realize the cognitive losses you have sustained. But when you are surrounded by people half your age — you feel every bit of the aging losses, physical and cognitively. That was my first experience of what my brain was able to accomplish when I pushed it hard.

The brain surgery was different because the losses were immediate and profound. I had knowledge of what brain health and brain function were all about. At that point I was grateful that I understood that I could change my brain. Looking back, it was amazing how the brain changes happened. It took belief and dedication to the process to make it happen.

Everything You Do Matters to Your Brain
Everything you do matters to your brain — good or bad. Do you sit around worrying about your weight while you are watching TV and munching on unhealthy snacks? Guess what — your brain won't like that. As your brain adapts to that environment you will feel sluggish, unhappy, stressed out. You can lose brain volume, have memory problems, not be as productive at work, not be interesting to your spouse, kids, or friends, and probably end up going to the doctor more often. If this is how you treat your brain, your brain will reciprocate.

Being Brain Fit

What does it look like when you are 'brain fit'? Brain fitness is that state of awareness that you are performing well cognitively and emotionally. You are running on all cylinders, maintaining a mental edge, staying sharp, aging successfully. Aging is a broad term in this context because our brain doesn't know how old we are. Your brain ages in response to lifestyle, chronic diseases, stress, and genes. So, your chronological age may be in the forties, but your brain age may be in the sixties because you live a hard life. You must take responsibility for how you live and the impact it makes on your brain.

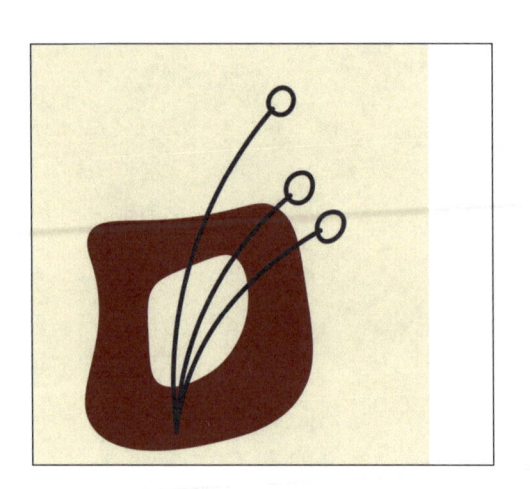

chapter three

What Are Brain Aging Losses?

Of course, I didn't think much about aging when I was younger. It never seemed like it was going to happen to me. Until it did! That was when the observational study of aging became real for me and added a whole new depth of understanding to what I am going through. Even though the aging brain is the focus of attention, it is important to flush out some ideas about the aging body. It does house our amazing brain and has a definite impact on how our brain functions.

The Aging Body
The aging process is tough, and there are so many changes occurring that we don't feel like we have any control over them. However, when we see the aging changes our body goes through, we realize that many of these changes are controllable.

As we age, our body goes through somewhat of a metamorphosis. We can see these changes occurring throughout the years, but we are still unnerved when we look in the mirror and that young fresh face is no longer looking back. The changes are gradual, and we don't pay attention and notice what is happening for years until we **see** the changes. We see gray hair, wrinkles, turkey neck, and jowls. Wrinkles and saggy skin drive a huge cosmetic market. It seems that our arms aren't long enough anymore to be able to read a menu without glasses. We start to experience weight gain in all the wrong places! None of us want to look old. As much as we don't want to admit it, we can't hear as well as when we were younger. Hearing loss is now considered an aging issue complete with isolation and cognitive decline. More serious changes that affect our body function include loss of flexibility, muscle strength, and decline in muscle mass. Our metabolism slows down and suddenly we feel OLD!

When you can see and accept physical aging and understand what is going on, it can spur you to make changes in your life to maintain a younger physical presence. The point I am trying to make is that we can see and understand that our body is aging. And we can make decisions on what we choose to do to maintain our youthful body and appearance. As a person gets older, changes occur in all parts of the body, including the brain. These are changes in an aging brain that we can't see.

- Certain parts of the brain shrink, especially those important to learning and other complex mental activities.
- In certain brain regions, communication between neurons (nerve cells) can be reduced.
- Blood flow in the brain may also decrease.
- Inflammation, which occurs when the body responds to an injury or disease, may increase.

The Aging Brain

Our brains age, just like our bodies. It happens to everyone whether you are a nuclear physicist, or you have never worked. Our brains shrink as we get older; neurons (brain cells) are dying in the regions of the prefrontal cortex and hippocampus. These areas are responsible for memory, learning, planning, and other complex mental tasks. Changes in our neurons and neurotransmitters (brain chemistry) affect communication between the cells in the brain. Therefore, we don't take in information and have a response as fast as when we were younger. This is called processing speed.

For me, it was a subtle change. A missed word, a lost name, a tip-of-the-tongue moment, and I was freaking out. What was happening to me? The kicker was the time I forgot a word in the middle of a presentation I had done at least ten times before. Sweat was rolling down my back, and many eyes were staring at me as I tried to talk around the word I forgot. FYI — I remembered that word about two hours later! That became a life-long memory and overshadowed every presentation I did from then on. My first reaction to this was "Lord have mercy! Was I in trouble? Was I experiencing the onset of dementia?"

Not content to sit in my fear, I started researching the workings of the aging brain. It was a bittersweet discovery that my brain was aging, and I was losing my quick-minded functioning. But I was not on the slippery slope to dementia. The moment that I discovered I could reverse these aging changes felt like a life-saving event to me.

What Happens When Our Brain Ages?

Let's start at the beginning of our brain journey. In the early years of life, the brain forms more than a million new neural connections **every second!** By the age of six, the size of the brain increases to about 90% of its volume in adulthood! Ultimately, at about three pounds of weight, the human brain is a staggering feat of engineering, with about **100 billion neurons** interconnected via **trillions of synapses**. (The places where neurons connect and communicate with each other.). Then in the 30s and 40s, the brain starts to shrink, with the shrinkage rate increasing even more by age 60. Although we can see the physical changes that are occurring with aging, we don't understand that our brain is also changing shape. That means that our cognitive abilities become altered.

These are the changes that happen:

- **Brain Mass**: While brain volume decreases overall with age, the frontal lobe and hippocampus — the area responsible for cognitive functions — shrink more than other areas of the brain.
- Frontal lobes — behind the forehead; largest lobes in the human brain; considered to be the human behavior and emotional control centers of personalities.
- The hippocampus — embedded deep within the temporal lobe; plays a major part in learning and memory.
- **Cortical Density**: This refers to the thinning of the outer corrugated surface of the brain due to decreasing synaptic connection.

- The cerebral cortex — the wrinkled outer layer of the brain that contains neuronal cell bodies is also thin with age.
- Lower density leads to fewer connections, which also contributes to slower cognitive processing.
- **White Matter**: Consists of myelinated nerve fibers that are bundled into tracts and transmit nerve signals between brain cells.
- Myelin shrinks with age, slowing down processing and reducing cognitive function.
- White matter is a vast, intertwining system of neural connections that join all four lobes of the brain (frontal, temporal, parietal, occipital), and the brain's emotional center in the limbic system.
- **Neurotransmitter System:** The brain begins to produce different levels of chemicals that affect neurotransmitters and protein production, ultimately leading to a decline in cognitive function. [1]

Why the neuroscience lesson? These changes have a major impact on brain function in older adults. This translates into these realities:

- Difficulty learning something new: Committing new information to memory can take longer.
- Multitasking: Slow processing can make planning parallel tasks more difficult.
- Recalling names and numbers: Strategic memory, which helps with remembering names and numbers, begins to decline at age 20.
- Remembering appointments: Without cues to recall

the information, the brain may put appointments into "storage" and not access them unless something jogs the person's memory.

This does sound dire, doesn't it? However, some positive changes occur with an aging brain. Older adults have more extensive vocabularies and greater knowledge of the depth of meaning of words than younger adults. Also, older adults may have learned from a lifetime of experiences and accumulated knowledge. In essence, older adults can still do many of the things they have enjoyed their whole lives:

- Learn new skills
- Form new memories
- Improve vocabulary and language skills [1]

But Wait! There Is More!

Through the recent research on neurogenesis and neuroplasticity, we now know that we can slow the brain aging process and increase brain volume as we get older. The brain's frontal cortex, which is used for problem-solving and some aspects of word processing, shrinks with age, but it also shows more activity as you get older. There is evidence that older adults can create new brain pathways to cope with diminished ones and to increase their processing capability (neuroplasticity).

Here is what is happening in our brains with certain aging slips:

- **Slow Processing Speed:**

Did you ever feel that your brain was unbelievably fast? You could give a response as soon as the last word is uttered? But now you must take a moment to "think" about what your response will be. Processing speed is the rate at which a person can take a new bit of information, reach some judgment on it, and formulate a response. In late middle age (40-60) our processing speed starts to decline at a slow and steady pace. Although the slowing of processing speed is not completely understood, the evidence does suggest that such a decline reflects wear and tear of the white matter of the brain, which is made up of all the wires, or axons, that connect one part of the brain to another. Slowed information transfer along axons may impede processing speed. [2]

- **Tip-of-the-Tongue Phenomenon:**

This is a very evident aging change and is very aggravating to experience. What is TOT all about? It is described by many sources as the failure to retrieve a word from memory. The left temporal and frontal areas of your brain have a communication breakdown. They don't work together to retrieve the words or names stored in long-term memory. You know the word you want; you can even remember the beginning letter; how many syllables the word has; or even how to stress the right part of the word. But no matter how hard you try — you can't recall the word in that moment.

There have been some studies focusing on TOT. Tip-of-the-tongue increases with age and during periods of stress. The brain doesn't like functioning when all the stress hormones are playing havoc with it. And it happens to most people at least once a week. (Good to know!) You have known this word for many years but cannot recall it at the moment you need it. The research studies have not determined why this happens. Long-term memories are stored within the memory system with memories that are accessible and available. Sometimes memories are inaccessible on a temporary or permanent basis. If the strength of the memory is not strong enough it becomes more difficult to recall the word, name, etc. There is some indication that the brain stores words and definitions in a way similar to a dictionary. Sometimes the more memories you need to go through to find that word can result in TOT.

- **Cognitive Flexibility:**

As we progress through our adult years, we count on the process of cognitive flexibility. You might not have known that you were practicing this skill when you had a lot going on and you had to make decisions based on a lot of different inputs. But you did! And now you are finding this skill out of your reach. Well, this is just another aging change.

Cognitive flexibility is the ability to switch between thinking about two different concepts or thinking about multiple concepts simultaneously. However, this mental flexibility declines with age, and juggling multiple streams of information needed for decision-making becomes more difficult the older you get. You don't excel at thinking on your feet when faced with a new situation. This realization is difficult to accept.

Our lifestyle determines what the impact of these changes will be on our brain. Genetics has about a 30% role in how our brain will age, but environment and lifestyle have a far greater impact on the brain. Do you lead a sedentary life, eat fatty foods, and watch TV all the time? OOPS — cognitive decline for you and a high risk of dementia! If you are active, eat nutritious meals, and challenge yourself mentally then you can lower your risk for dementia. Our brains are very adaptable and constantly changing to our environment. Our brain is also an energy cannibal – this three-pound organ uses 20% of blood, oxygen, and glucose from each heartbeat. If you provide this environment for your brain, you can offset the aging changes taking place. Your brain can grow new brain cells in the hippocampus, which is the center of learning and memory. You also increase the flow of neurotransmitters and help facilitate communication within your brain. You will be helping your brain continue to function at its highest level.

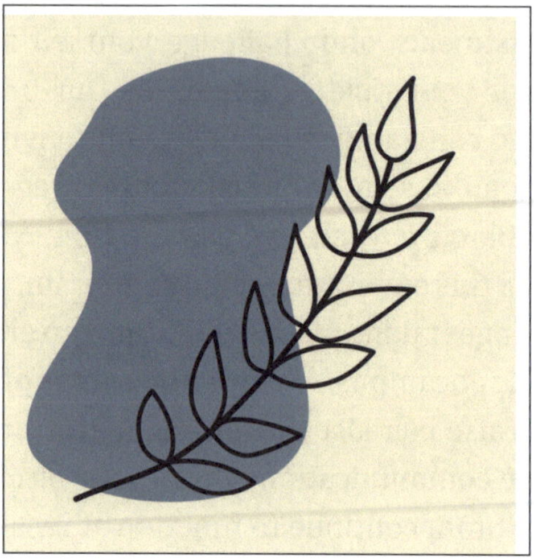

chapter four

When Science Found the Fountain of Youth

I went back to grad school when I was fifty years old. My classmates were twenty-five! I didn't think much about the age difference because I was just happy to be continuing my education. However, that age difference made a huge impact within the first couple of weeks of school. Grad school moves fast. There is no waiting around for everyone to be on the same page. School has always been my thing though, and I didn't think I would have any trouble doing the work. Was I ever wrong! One example of this age difference came when we were in class and the professor was asking some questions about an assignment. My classmates were shouting out the answers while I was trying to figure out what the professor was asking. I was like a deer in headlights! What had I done to myself? What happened next was a miracle created by my brain.

It was very hard work, but I pushed my brain to work better and remember more. This involved being super prepared for every class. To do this I had to commit more concentrated time to doing the classwork. When the reading was long, I just stuck with it until I finished. I also took lots of notes as I read so that the important information would be at my disposal. Even learning how to research on a computer was a huge challenge for me. *Little did I know at that time, I was creating a younger more vibrant brain.*

What happens in the brain to generate new neurons and synaptic connections? Here is the secret sauce!

NEUROGENESIS

Every time I hear the word neurogenesis, the soundtrack for 2001 A Space Odyssey pops into my head. The difference is the movie was science fiction and neurogenesis is grounded in science. Neurogenesis is the birth of brain cells. Up until about thirty years ago this concept of growing new brain cells was considered science fiction. The consensus over the years was that the brain we had around age twenty-five would be as good as it gets. From that age, we couldn't create new brain cells and our brain would decline until the day we died! In 1998, researchers confirmed that regeneration of new neurons did occur in certain areas of the brain. This regeneration of new brain cells is called neurogenesis and is the ability of the adult brain to produce immature neurons in the mature human brain. There was much doubt that a confirmed finding of neurogenesis in an adult brain would ever be discovered. When imaging studies became more sophisticated, photos of new neural stem cells were seen budding in the hippocampus, the center of learning and memory. This was a huge discovery and changed the way we thought about the brain forever.

What do we need to do to create new brain cells? This answer works for everyone! It all comes down to physical exercise.

The prefrontal cortex (the area behind the forehead) is an energy cannibal because it is the executive function center of the brain. Being the main player in brain function it requires a lot of energy. Because the brain doesn't have its energy source, it requires 20% of carbohydrates, oxygen, and blood from each heartbeat for it to function. If you live a sedentary life and spend your days sitting in front of a computer or maybe a TV, your brain is lethargic. It does not have the energy it needs to do to maintain its high-functioning capacity.

There must be an initiator for the process of neurogenesis to happen. The increased surge of blood, oxygen, and carbohydrates from exercise releases an important growth factor called brain-derived neurotrophic factor, (BDNF). BDNF acts as a fertilizer for the brain because it stimulates the budding of neuron stem cells and protects these young cells as they mature. BDNF is also responsible for the growth of new neurons that replace the losses we sustain as we grow older. The prefrontal cortex and the hippocampus take the biggest hits in cell loss. But they are also the two areas where neurogenesis has been documented to occur. Exercise stimulates neurogenesis – the creation of new neurons – primarily in the hippocampus, influencing memory and learning.

NEUROPLASTICITY

Talking to people who only believe what they can see, taste, touch, smell, and feel can be very frustrating. Because they don't understand scientific research, they tend to deny the outcomes of this research. So, how can you get someone to understand that their brain is magnificent, and they can change their brain?

In the 1990s, research started coming forth that our brains had more adaptive power than we ever imagined.

Dr. Michael Merzenich, considered the Father of Neuroplasticity, was one of the most influential researchers in neuroplasticity in the early 1970s. The accepted hypothesis at the time was that the brain was compartmentalized, specialized, and fixed. He also believed that the brain could not change. What he discovered, however, was that the brain is constantly changing by learning and relearning. When one area of the brain is damaged, another area can relearn to function. This was a profound discovery. The process is neuroplasticity — the ability of the brain to adapt to its environment — good or bad. As we have already discussed, neurogenesis is the growth of new brain cells. Through these two processes, we can start to replace the brain mass that we are losing as we get older. You can create a healthy, resilient brain through neuroplasticity and neurogenesis.

Our brain does not know how old we are. If our life is toxic, meaning full of chronic stress and bad lifestyle habits, our brains will age faster by losing greater numbers of neurons and neural pathways. We put ourselves at a higher risk of developing dementia. But, if we lead a healthy lifestyle in a novel and complex environment, we continue to grow new neurons and neural pathways leading to a younger, high-functioning brain. We can create an ageless brain.

Our brain can change and rewire itself in response to the stimulation of learning and lifestyle circumstances. If you focus on something repetitively and consistently, that signal becomes stronger creating a new neuronal pathway. You have rewired your brain. The combination of neurogenesis and neuroplasticity can change our brains. We have the power to prevent Alzheimer's and maintain a high-functioning brain for our entire life.

The early pioneers in the discovery and function of neurogenesis and neuroplasticity have written extraordinary books to describe the impact of our ability to change our brains. Dr. Norman Doidge captured stories of personal triumph from neuroplasticity in his book, *"The Brain that Changes Itself,"* a New York Times bestseller. This book was revolutionary at the time of its publication.

"Doidge's book is a remarkable and hopeful portrait of the endless adaptability of the human brain... Only a few decades ago, scientists considered the brain to be fixed or 'hardwired,' and considered most forms of brain damage, therefore, to be incurable. Dr. Doidge, an eminent psychiatrist and researcher, was struck by how his patients' transformations belied this and set out to explore the new science of neuroplasticity by interviewing both scientific pioneers in neuroscience and patients who benefited from neurorehabilitation. Here he describes in fascinating personal narratives how the brain, far from being fixed, has remarkable powers of changing its structure and compensating for even the most challenging neurological conditions.

"Oliver Sacks (Oliver Sacks was a pioneer in the discovery of neuroplasticity. His book, *'The Man Who Thought His Wife Was a Hat'* is one of the classics in neuroscience research.)

I want to bring you the "best of the best" information about neurogenesis and neuroplasticity. There is no one better than Dr. Michael Merzenich.

"One of the foremost researchers of neuroplasticity, Dr. Michael Merzenich's work has shown that the brain retains its ability to alter itself well into adulthood – suggesting that brains with injuries or disease might be able to recover function even later in life." [3]

Dr. Merzenich authored *Soft-Wired, How the New Science of Brain Plasticity Can Change Your Life.* The father of neuroplasticity takes many case studies of people with various brain issues and weaves a story of recovery through the power of neuroplasticity. One of his most prolific topics is how the aging brain can change itself. What previously was an inconceivable idea, Dr. Merzenich teaches us how neuroplasticity can give us the gift of a younger brain. Capturing the power of neuroplasticity in a way that is understandable to nonscientists is one of Dr. Merzenich's strongest skills. If you want to get a clearer picture of how neuroplasticity can change your life, then *Soft-Wired* is a must-read.

Our brain determines who we are and how we function. Our brain only functions on a high level in the later years because of the lifestyle that we lead. What does that mean for you and me? My aging brain terrified me before I knew what was happening. However, the newer research into neurogenesis and neuroplasticity offered me hope that I could turn things around. Understanding how our brain sustains losses as we age empowers us to make life changes to create a sharper brain. These discoveries offer us the fountain of youth! You hold the power to change your brain. Think about it! You can turn your aging brain around and regain the vibrant brain you used to have! This can change your life and you can do it.

Strategic Plan to Reclaim Your Brain

Now, your brain is very cool! You treat it better, and it will respond to that. If you make a strategic plan to reclaim your brain, your brain will respond —that is the beauty of neuroplasticity. It requires concentrated effort, however. You cannot be complacent about your brain and must firmly believe that you can create new neural pathways and grow new brain cells. But you must be all in – not wishy-washy about it. Repetition and consistency create new neural pathways. This is where a brain-healthy lifestyle (physical exercise, mental stimulation, nutrition, socialization, sleep, and stress reduction) all play an important part. When you put the effort in to build a better brain, you will experience better health overall. Again, it doesn't make any difference what your age is. It is totally up to you and your commitment.

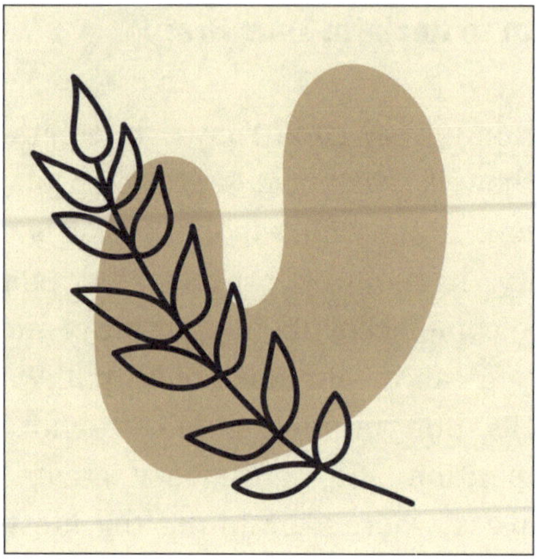

chapter five

This Sounds Too Good to Be True!

I get excited when I talk about brain aging and brain health. What wasn't so obvious was the fear I experienced with brain aging changes and feeling totally out of control over what was happening.

Throughout my entire life, I was blessed to have a high-functioning brain and I counted on it to function on a very high level. So, when I first learned about regaining my younger brain, I was over the moon. At that time, though, it was more on an intellectual level. I was learning, but not yet fully immersed in a brain-healthy lifestyle. However, in 2012, I had brain surgery. I have Meniere's disease which is a build-up of fluid in the chambers of the inner ear. Meniere's is devastating. It can cause vertigo, nausea, ringing in the ears, and/or headache. I had all these symptoms. The problems started in 2003, while I was in grad school. Trust me, it was hard for me to function normally when I was this sick. I lost 40 pounds over the next nine years, had three ear surgeries, and fell a few times too many. My biggest concern was that people would think I was drunk because I could not walk in a straight line. When I walked into the grocery store or hardware store, I thought I was going to fall. If you have ever fallen in a public location, you might have suffered through the embarrassment of people staring at you. It was not an enriching experience. A cart was always necessary to hold on to because clutching the handle kept me upright. What a nightmare that was. Finally, I was scheduled for a Vestibular Nerve Section. *The vestibular system functions to detect the position and movement of our head in space.* It allows for the coordination of eye movements, posture, and equilibrium. The inner ear houses the vestibular system and helps to accomplish these tasks by sending nerve signals from its components.

My Brain-Changing Event

My vestibular system wasn't working. Testing revealed that the right side of my brain had only 15% balance function while the left side maintained 100% balance function. My brain could not reconcile the difference between the large gap in balance function. Balance rehab at that point made my situation worse. The only step left was to have the vestibular nerve section performed. This surgery clipped the vestibular nerve at the brain stem on the right side so that no nerve signals would get to my brain.

I had no idea what to expect. A few weeks before the surgery I received an offer to speak about brain health scheduled shortly after the surgery. I had to call my doctor to see if I could accept the offer! The answer was a resounding "no". The surgery lasted for five hours, and I was under deep anesthesia. The lengthy anesthesia proved to be a problem with my recovery because of severe brain fog. There was no pain associated with this surgery, but not being able to think was unnerving! Recovery from brain fog had to happen immediately for me to feel better and have the stamina to go through the physical rehab. Since I knew about brain health, I knew how to put a brain health program together for me. My immediate effort was to find a brain game application that helped me regain focus, attention, speed of processing, and recall. At that time, I found an online ten-minute daily program that started helping with my speed of processing and focus. It didn't wear me out and I could see some progress quickly. Every day I met tougher challenges that pushed my brain to recover. This brain rehab lasted for at least nine months. It was then I felt clear enough to stay focused on my physical rehab and continue to stay involved with cognitive exercises.

After the surgery, I had NO balance function on the right side of my brain. I couldn't stand, my head would swim when I moved it, and I was an extremely high fall risk. It was discouraging to be in that kind of condition. A month after surgery I was scheduled for balance rehab. I had to learn to walk and move without feeling like I was going to fall.

Now here comes the good part. The rehab lasted eight weeks and the exercises involved not only moving but also retraining my eye movement. The vestibular system is composed of the eyes, inner ear, and brain. It was hard and progress was slow but there was progress. My rehab homework was intense; and if I didn't do my exercises every day, I would backslide. To make a change in your brain you must practice an exercise repetitively and consistently. When you do that, you are sending new signals to the brain and starting the process of creating new synaptic connections. The ultimate goal was to have the left side of my brain take over all balance functions. And it did! Little did I know that it would take so long. In the end, it was three years before I felt like I was almost normal again. The brain is a miraculous gift. It can change and give you your life back, but you must do the work to make that happen.

Debbie Hampton. Founder of The Best Brain Possible and Brain-Changer

To demonstrate how neuroplasticity can change your life, I need to introduce you to my friend, Debbie Hampton. I met Debbie through a couple of brain-related masterminds. These were meetings where everyone had special knowledge about brain function. This was the time I experienced accelerated knowledge about brain health. Debbie is the founder of "The Best Brain Possible." Her story is one of tragedy and then recovery. Her memoir *Sex, Suicide and Serotonin* chronicles her journey to recovery after emerging from a week-long coma. Debbie had attempted to "end her life." The difference from other attempts was this time she almost succeeded. She had swallowed a handful of pills seven days earlier and the consequences were horrific: a massive traumatic brain injury, she couldn't speak: words were garbled, speech was slow, and she couldn't control the volume of her speech. Debbie recounted that she had to learn how to perform the basics of living again: breathing, swallowing, eating, controlling her bladder, and communicating. It seemed inconceivable to her at that time that her life would ever be manageable again.

Debbie had intense physical, occupational, and speech

therapy as part of her initial recovery stage. In her words "After ten weeks of outpatient therapy, it was scary as hell to hear the neurologist say, 'Well, all we can do at this point is wait and see.' All I knew then was that it felt pretty darn shitty not to be told of anything I could be doing to improve."

Over the next year, she did improve naturally by getting lots of rest and doing the everyday things that life requires. But nearly a year post-injury she plateaued with impaired mental processing, unreliable short-term memory, and disjointed thoughts and speech.

She thought, "There HAS got to be something else I can do. I'm NOT staying this way. If I am going to live, it sure as hell isn't going to be like this!"

With the lifting of her brain fog, she was able to investigate every bit of information that might lead to something that might help her. She began doing everything she could independently to improve. Her initial discovery was that the more she did, the better she got. And the better she got, the more she did. So, what did she do?

One of Debbie's friends introduced her to Bikram Yoga. This particular yoga practice is 90 minutes of Hatha yoga in a room heated to 105 degrees. The intense heat increases flexibility decreases the risk of injury and allows a person to rework their body. Improved balance, coordination, and breathwork helped Debbie learn to breathe while talking. The brain benefits from retraining the brain in response to stress in the body.

Neurofeedback was the next therapeutic practice she investigated to reclaim her brain. Neurofeedback is a specialized form of biofeedback for the brain in which a person's body learns to alter their brainwaves. The learning occurs at a subconscious level and results in permanent physical changes in the brain. Neurofeedback is not a one-time-only experience. You are rewiring your brain; so again, repetition and consistency are critical. For Debbie, after the first ten sessions, she experienced her speech and thoughts come together. Sleep became deeper and more restful, allowing her brain to make some serious healing. With her frontal lobe functioning optimally, her emotions stabilized, and she became calmer and more positive. She regained mental stamina, accomplished more, and her life became easier. After a year and a half of neurofeedback therapy, Debbie felt almost completely normal again. This may seem like a long time, but Debbie was rewiring her brain to attain a normal functioning brain again. Neuroplasticity is growing new brain pathways and processes — like a baby's neuronal growth. This is neuroplasticity at its finest. Debbie had tapped into the power of her brain to change to come back from a catastrophic brain injury.

However, this success led her to discover other alternative therapies that would continue the work of healing her brain. The next healing modality she tried was acupuncture. Her first appointment delivered profound results in her perception. She describes it as if the lens she was looking through at life was refocused. For the next few years, she did cranial acupuncture. Needles were placed all over her head and attached via clips and wires to a machine that sent electrical impulses into them to provide stimulation. She was recharging her brain! Debbie continued acupuncture long after she recovered from her brain injury for wellness support and various aches and pains she experienced.

One other therapy Debbie employed during her recovery was Hyperbaric Oxygen Therapy (HBOT). In HBOT therapy, a person is exposed to increased atmospheric pressure in a room or inflatable chamber, permitting them to breathe pure oxygen at a higher level than found naturally in the atmosphere. The extra pressure allows a person's blood to dissolve up to ten times more oxygen, which not only increases the oxygen in the blood, but also permits it to pass into tissue, cells, and the brain more easily. After continued HBOT treatments, the tissues of the body are permanently changed. Debbie related that she experienced substantial healing on all fronts, but the most dramatic benefit was mental.

"Like the sun bursting from behind the clouds, my brain fog cleared and the invisible veil of the brain injury that separated me from the rest of the world evaporated as I returned to full consciousness. I've continued HBOT over the years, as maintenance and still feel it working its magic. If I go too long in between sessions, my speech suffers - but improves immediately after time in the chamber."

Debbie went on to incorporate many different physical practices into her life - running, swimming, dancing, jumping rope. These were must-dos every day for four and a half years. At that time, she felt that she had recovered enough to get back to the art of living. Today, if you didn't know what Debbie's journey entailed, you would never know that she had experienced a traumatic brain injury. Her years of pushing her brain to recover are an inspiration to me and fully demonstrate the power of neuroplasticity to change and regain our brain.

It is important to remember that neuroplasticity is a double-edged sword. What you focus on is the way you change your brain. It can be for the positive or the negative. What does that mean? You have just read how Debbie and I changed our brains with the positive focus of healing. Our brains responded in kind. But what happens when you see, hear, and experience the negative side of life constantly? Your brain will reinforce those negative feelings and you can end up miserable. Negative emotions and negative thinking will get etched into your brain and rule your life. You will experience physical ramifications from this stress including many chronic diseases that are the result of systemic inflammation. Heart disease, diabetes, arthritis, gastrointestinal problems, and auto-immune diseases put you at a higher risk of dementia. Neuroplasticity can also help you prevent the onset of dementia. A complex positive environment will challenge your brain to rewire itself.

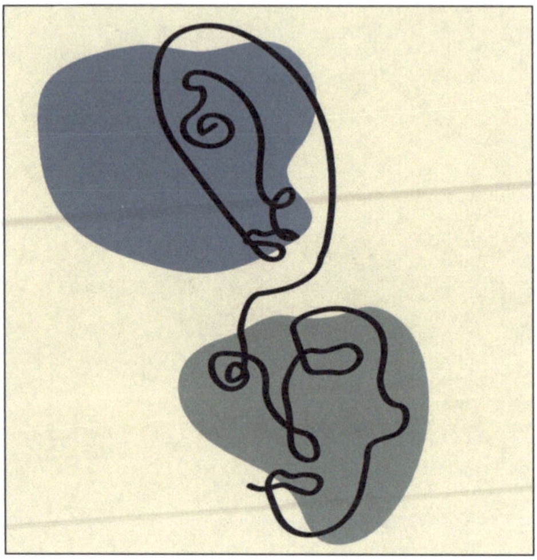

chapter six

COVID: A Stress Test for Your Brain

What if your aging brain has taken a beating throughout your life? What happens when your brain has been the recipient of a more toxic lifestyle? Can you still change your brain?

There was no better example of a difficult lifestyle situation than what we all experienced with the COVID-19 pandemic. My goodness, what a mess we were all thrown into. Fear of the unknown was the initial response. How can we battle a virus we cannot see?

Besides the fear of getting a potentially fatal disease, you had to deal with all the emotions associated with losing your job and subsequent income. If you have never been in a situation like this before — it can devastate you. Your bills don't end, your health can take a hit, and your brain stays stuck in a chronic stress loop. At this point, you can't even think. Your brain has been hijacked by the flooding of cortisol and incoming information completely bypasses your prefrontal cortex — the executive function center of your brain. The prefrontal cortex makes your decisions, does your planning, and is the center of conscious thought. When you are in stress mode, the prefrontal cortex is eliminated from the thinking process. Now all incoming signals are going directly to the amygdala, the emotional center of the brain. Instead of thinking through a problem, the amygdala orchestrates an emotional reaction. So instead of thinking, you are reacting. This is not a viable strategy to be able to handle all the crises that are occurring in your life.

And the Stress Goes On and On and On

Something is exciting about the start of a crisis. Your brain automatically goes into fight or flight and releases adrenalin. Your body is primed for survival – your senses are sharp and physically you feel like you can take on anything that comes your way.

But then, when the stressors don't stop, your life is turned upside down, and thrown into places where you have never been. You aren't working and have no income, yet there are bills to pay and food to buy. The stressors are escalating faster than your ability to solve your problems.

Your brain has now changed. Instead of using your prefrontal cortex (area of the brain behind your forehead) to think, plan, and make decisions; you have created a loop between your hippocampus and amygdala (emotional center of the brain). Now you are reacting, rather than thinking. Emotions have taken over, creating worry and anxiety. You can't eat; you can't sleep; and everyone is on your last nerve. Cortisol, the stress hormone, is flooding your brain and body. This is one destructive hormone; it even kills brain cells. On top of everything else – now your brain is shrinking!

Okay — time to take a breath. Your brain has been on automatic pilot to help you survive. The problem is — our threat alert and survival system were created to keep our prehistoric ancestors alive, not find your way through a long-lasting pandemic. We do have control over our brain function or the thoughts that pop into our heads. They are generated by our subconscious brain. We have control over which ones we believe in and act on. In this circumstance we had to be open to learning a new skill set; one that would allow us to calm down, get centered, and start thinking again. One way to do this is to calm your breathing. When you take three deep breaths, you can reset your nervous system. Breathe in through your nose on a count of four. Your belly should be extending on this inhalation. Hold your breath to a count of seven. Then exhale through your pursed lips to a count of eight. Your belly should be going down on the exhale. Keep your attention on your breathing. This simple exercise has the power to break the chronic stress loop.

When you get out of bed in the morning, make an intention to trust yourself. Saying affirmations like this can help: "As I heal and grow, it will all work out." "Relax and trust me." Say something similar every morning before you start your day. Your problems won't disappear but now they are more controllable because you are using your brain again.

If you find that you can't focus on these different activities because you are still worried, then you need to look at other options to calm your brain. You could take the time to journal your experiences through this ordeal. Don't read your entry from yesterday before you write your new entry. The purpose of journaling is to get some of the stress and frustration out and on paper. When you see your written words, you may see solutions pop up too. When you get to a point where you are resuming as normal a life as you can, you can go back and read your story. Then honor the progress you made in retraining your brain.

Your emotional response to the stressors of COVID changed your brain. The environment was toxic, and your brain adapted to the difficult situations you were facing. Your brain took a hit; cells were lost; emotions went uncontrolled.

Then there was the physical toll our brain sustained from COVID. Research results were being made public about a year into the pandemic. What was the primary site for infection? This was considered primarily a respiratory virus. However, the research painted a more complex, serious pathway of infection. Dr. Gabriel de Erausquin, researcher at UT Health San Antonio, published a study along with his colleagues, including senior author Dr. Sudha Seshadri, a professor of neurology at UT Health San Antonio and director of the University's Glenn Biggs Institute for Alzheimer's and Neurodegenerative Diseases. [4] Their basic premise was that the respiratory viruses have an affinity for nervous system cells. Prof. Seshadri explains, "Olfactory cells are very susceptible to viral invasion and are particularly targeted by SARS-CoV-2, and that is why one of the prominent symptoms of COVID-19 is loss of smell."

Olfactory cells are concentrated in the nose. Through these cells, the virus reaches the olfactory bulb in the brain, which is located near the hippocampus, the center of learning and memory.

"The trail of the virus, when it invades the brain, leads almost straight to the hippocampus," explains Dr. de Erausquin. "That is believed to be one of the sources of cognitive impairment observed in COVID-19 patients. We suspect it may also be part of the reason why there will be an accelerated cognitive decline over time in susceptible individuals." [5]

What Ways Does Coronavirus Affect the Brain?

Cases around the world show that patients with COVID-19 can have a variety of conditions related to the brain, including:

- Confusion
- Loss of consciousness
- Seizures
- Stroke
- Loss of smell and taste
- Headaches
- Trouble focusing
- Changes in behavior

Patients are also having peripheral nerve issues, such as Guillain-Barre syndrome, which can lead to paralysis and respiratory failure. [6]

Potential Outcomes of COVID-19 Infection

The brain is one of the regions where viruses like to hide. Unlike the lungs, the brain is not as equipped, from an immunological perspective to clear viruses. That's why we're seeing severe disease and all these multiple symptoms like heart disease, stroke, and all these long haulers with loss of smell, and loss of taste. All of this has to do with the brain, rather than the lungs. [5]

Senior Researcher Kumar cautions that the brain damage may mean that many people with COVID-19 continue to be at a high risk of neurodegenerative diseases, such as Parkinson's, multiple sclerosis, or general cognitive decline, after recovering. Unfortunately, it appears that many people who have COVID-19 will face a very uncertain cognitive future. [5]

Writing this makes my blood run cold. When I first researched this subject, I had been vaxed and boosted and was feeling good. Then I tested COVID positive in September 2022. I felt pretty good for a couple of weeks after a negative test result. But then I started coughing and I coughed every day and night for four months! I couldn't even talk without coughing. There was severe fatigue, continued loss of taste and smell, trouble focusing, and brain fog. The group of long-hauler COVID sufferers now included me! Initially, I was too sick to be concerned. Time kept moving by and I wasn't recovering. I felt the fear of never being well again. That is an emotional statement, but the losses I have sustained since getting sick leave me depressed. My lungs are scarred, and I now have a pulmonologist overseeing my lung care. The brain fog is horrific! It is impossible to keep up the schedule of writing, speaking, and working that I was accustomed to. There are two online magazines I submit articles to, and I asked for a leave of absence because I couldn't put two words together. The apprehension over the losses from an aging brain pales in comparison to the fear I am experiencing right now. After all, my brain is "my thing." So, what now?

I accepted the fact that my brain needs a lot of work. It is time to double down on the brain-healthy lifestyle (see Chapter Eight). Recently I subscribed to Posit Science Brainhq. Although it is referred to as brain games, I find that it works as brain rehab for me. The exercises target focus, attention, memory, and speed of processing, among other specific brain functions. Targeting these specific functions allows the magic of neuroplasticity to begin and rewire my brain. I refuse to let cognitive decline define me.

Brain Resilience

It is not the strongest of the species that survived, nor the most intelligent that survives. It is the one that is most adaptable to change.

Charles Darwin

It is important to me to write about brain resilience at this point. Aging is not for sissies! Everything changes as we age. Our health and normal physical aging changes might throw us for a loop. We sustain losses of family, friends, husbands, and wives. And the lives we are living now might not ever return to their status quo since the pandemic.

Stress and Resilience

Resilience is a process of your brain adapting to significant stress, adversity, trauma, tragedy, or threats. Our brain is hardwired to protect us by automatically going into a stress response mode. Throughout human history, we have had to be resilient to survive. The autonomic nervous system (ANS) is responsible for all automatic functions without conscious thought, such as breathing, regulating heart rate, and digestive processes. The ANS is basic to resilience because it keeps us in a "window of tolerance." So, we are made to develop resilience. We don't have to figure it out or learn what to do – we are hard-wired to withstand the big blows of life. As it turns out, our brain plays a role in bouncing back/resilience by determining how we react to challenging circumstances and guiding us in recovery.

The stress response happens below our level of awareness and a cascade of stress chemicals are released before we are even aware that our brain is responding. Although this was a necessary reaction for our ancestors to stay alive, we live in a very different world. There is a feedback loop that will stop the acute stress response; but because we are living in a 24/7 information overload society, our brains may feel like they are being threatened. Instead of resetting, our brain goes into a chronic stress cycle. The Hypothalamic – Pituitary – Adrenal axis is activated and now cortisol (the stress hormone) is released. An ongoing overabundance of cortisol kills brain cells. It also instigates other physical changes that can damage our health and possibly our lives. At this point, your brain starts to rise to the occasion or sink to the situation. This is where resilience comes into play. So, if we are hard-wired to develop resilience, why do some people never recover? Bear with me as I explain a little more about our miraculous brains. The Prefrontal Cortex (PFC) is the executive function center of the brain. The PFC ends the fear response, regulates emotions, learns, and exercises empathy, and exhibits response flexibility — the process of resilience. Finally, it is the PFC that creates the narrative of our lives. The ability to bounce back comes from our brain. And our brain learns from experience whenever we encounter a tough situation. This is a possible explanation as to why some people can bounce back, and others can't. As miraculous as our brains are, it still adapts to our environment — good or bad. The experience of hard times or challenging situations teaches our brains to handle tougher situations. Even though we have the brain anatomy to survive and bounce back, we are still human, and we always interject our subjective response to the situation. Learning to trust our intuition will help develop resilience and allow us to recover.

Resilience is not an automatic response to significant stress. It is a learned response that offers hope for those who are buried in the chronic stress cycle. Because resilience is a learned response, it is a process of neuroplasticity. This means that if you learn to bounce back from chronic stress, you will change your brain to be able to recover from life's challenges.

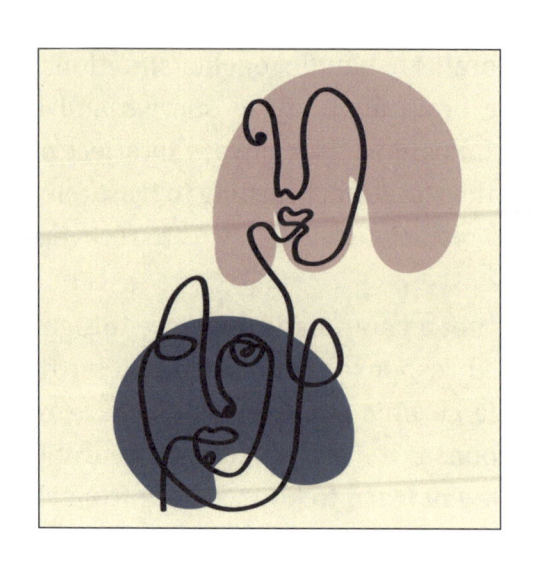

chapter seven

Brain Health Challenges for Boomers and Everyone Else

Reflect on your past. What kind of lifestyle have you led? Was it easy and stress-free or have you had to battle to get through each day? Granted, none of us have an either/or in this scenario. We live our lives and adjust as we go. But when you get to your older years, you are the sum of all those life habits and experiences. What risk factors for dementia are we looking at when we hit our senior years?

Over the past fifteen years, I have been researching and learning about brain aging and health. One of the terms that is thrown around consistently is "risk factor." It has been a go-to term in my blogs and speaking engagements when I am talking about dementia. In writing about chronic disease's impact on the brain, I finally learned what risk factors mean.

Risk Factors are aspects of your lifestyle, environment, and genetic background that increase a person's chances of developing a condition. Some risk factors cannot be avoided:

Non-modifiable Risk Factors

- **Age** – Dementia is not a normal part of aging, but age is the strongest known risk factor for developing dementia. This means that a person who is aged over 75 is more likely to develop dementia than someone under 75. The older you get, your chances of developing dementia increase.
- **Sex** – Women are at a higher risk of developing dementia and Alzheimer's disease than men. Potential contributors to this include:

    Women live longer (on average) than men.

    Changes in estrogen levels over a woman's lifetime.
- **Genetics** – Although the role of genetics in the development of dementia is not fully understood, scientists have found over 20 genes that may increase the risk of developing Alzheimer's disease. Even though genetics is a non-modifiable risk factor, it has two different types of genes that determine if you will develop dementia or be at a high risk of developing dementia.

Deterministic genes:

- Of the twenty genes that are associated with Alzheimer's disease, three genes directly **cause** Alzheimer's disease – PS1, PS2, and APP.
- If a person has an alteration in any of these genes, they will almost certainly develop familial Alzheimer's, often well before the age of 65. However, familial Alzheimer's disease is very rare.
- If a parent has any of these faulty genes, their children

have a 50% chance of inheriting the disease.

Risk Factor genes:

- The other 17 genes associated with Alzheimer's disease are called "risk factor" genes, meaning that the genes increase the risk, but do not guarantee the person will develop Alzheimer's. (Risk Factors, Alzheimer's Society)

Modifiable Risk Factors

These are the risk factors we have control over and can change. Cardiovascular disease has a very strong link to dementia. High blood pressure, high cholesterol levels, diabetes, stroke, and heart disease can all increase your risk.

Your lifestyle determines how fast your brain ages. Unhealthy lifestyle choices can accelerate brain aging, meaning that you will lose cell volume faster. This is the current list of modifiable risk factors. I will review the effects of each of these lifestyle choices so that you can see how they damage your brain and increase your risk for dementia.

- **Smoking:** It seems to put you at risk for dementia, possibly because it is bad for your blood vessels. It makes you more likely to have a stroke, which can and often does damage the brain and cause vascular dementia. This might lead to problems with thinking or remembering. Talk to your doctor or a mental health professional if you smoke and want support to quit. (WebMD. Medically reviewed by Carol Sarlissian, MD. (May 27, 2022). Things that raise your chances of dementia.)

- **Chronic Alcohol Use:** Regularly drinking above the recommended amounts of alcohol exposes the brain to higher levels of toxic substances that can damage nerve cells over time. The recommended amount of alcohol per week is two drinks a day for men, and one drink a day for women. This should be spread out over at least three days rather than one. (Alzheimer's Society. (June 2021). Risk factors for dementia. https://www.alzheimers.org.uk) [8]

- **Low Levels of Cognitive Engagement:** Cognitive engagement is thought to support the development of "cognitive reserve." This is the idea that people who actively use their brains throughout their lives may be more protected against brain cell damage caused by dementia. This means people with larger cognitive reserves can delay the start of dementia symptoms for a longer period. People with a smaller cognitive reserve are at a higher risk of getting dementia in their lifetime.

The three most important factors that can lead to a smaller cognitive reserve are:

1. Leaving education early: a person who left school at an early age is more likely to have a smaller cognitive reserve than a person who stayed in full-time education for longer or who continued throughout their life.

2. Less job complexity: a person who has not used a range of mental skills during their lifetime of work – for example, memory, reasoning, problem-solving, communication, and organizational skills – is more likely to have a smaller cognitive reserve.

3. Social isolation: a person who has not interacted much with other people during their life may also have a smaller cognitive reserve. (Alzheimer's Society. (June 2021). Risk factors for dementia. https://www.alzheimers.org.uk) [8]

- **Obesity and Lack of Physical Exercise:** Obesity in midlife (ages 45-65) increases your risk of developing dementia. Physical inactivity can worsen the health of a person's heart, lungs, and blood circulation, and make it harder for them to control their blood sugar. It is closely linked to a higher risk of heart disease, stroke, and type 2 diabetes, which are all risk factors for dementia. (Alzheimer's Society. (June 2021). Risk factors for dementia. https://www.alzheimers.org.uk) [8]
- **Social Isolation/Loneliness:** Social isolation can increase the risk of hypertension, coronary artery disease, depression, and dementia. Feeling lonely over time can increase your chances of having dementia, even when your overall risk of getting the disease — such as with genetics or age — is low, a 10-year study found. People under age 80 who reported feeling alone were twice as likely to have dementia as those who didn't feel that way. Time is key, though. People who recovered from their loneliness didn't have the same risk. Staying socially active may also help slow down the progression of the disease. (WebMD. Medically reviewed by Carol Sarlissian, MD. (May 27, 2022). Things that raise your chances of dementia.) [7]
- **Poor Diet:** Eating a diet that lacks a good range of healthy foods may increase a risk of dementia. There are many possible reasons. For example, an unhealthy

diet increases the risk of high blood pressure which is a risk factor for dementia. Ideally, a person should eat lots of fruits and vegetables, whole grain cereals, fish, healthy fats, dairy, and beans, and not too much red meat or processed food. Too much salt (more than a teaspoon a day) is also linked with a higher risk of dementia.

(Alzheimer's Society. (June 2021). Risk factors for dementia. https://www.alzheimers.org.uk) [8]

- **Diabetes:** Doctors aren't sure why people with diabetes get dementia more often. However, they do know that people with diabetes are more likely to have damaged blood vessels. This can slow or block blood flow to the brain and damage areas of the brain, leading to what's called vascular dementia. Some people may be able to slow brain decline if they keep diabetes under control with medicine, exercise, and a healthy diet. (WebMD. Medically reviewed by Carol Sarlissian, MD. (May 27, 2022). Things that raise your chances of dementia.). [7]

- **Hypertension:** People who have consistently high blood pressure in midlife (45-65) are more likely to develop vascular dementia. Vascular dementia is the second most common form of dementia after Alzheimer's disease. It is caused by reduced blood flow to the brain, which starves brain cells of the oxygen they need to function correctly. (Alzheimer's Society. High blood pressure and dementia. https://www.alzheimer's.org.uk/about-dementia/risk-factors-and-prevention/high-blood-pressure) [9]

- **Traumatic Brain Injury:** A single, mild traumatic

brain injury may not make you more likely to get dementia later in life. But more severe or repeated hits or falls could double or quadruple your chances, even years after the first injury. Get to the hospital if you have hit your head and you pass out, have blurry vision, or feel dizzy, confused, nauseated, or become sensitive to light. (WebMD. Medically reviewed by Carol Sarlissian, MD. (May 27, 2022). Things that raise your chances of dementia.) [7]

- **Hearing Loss:** Hearing loss can make the brain work harder, forcing it to strain to hear and fill in the gaps. That comes at the expense of other thinking and memory systems. Hearing loss causes the aging brain to shrink more quickly! One more contributing factor: Hearing loss leads people to be less socially engaged, which is hugely important to remain intellectually stimulated. (John Hopkins Bloomberg School of Public Health. (November 12, 2021). Hearing loss and the dementia connection. https://publichealth.jhu.edu/2012/hearing-loss-and-the-dementia-connection) [10]

- **Depression:** If you have depression, or have had it in the past, you may be more likely to get dementia. Scientists aren't yet sure that is a cause. It may simply be an early symptom or a sign of other causes like Parkinson's disease or Huntington's disease. Talk to your doctor or a therapist if you feel down for more than two weeks, and right away if you think of harming yourself. Therapy and medication can help with depression. (WebMD. Medically reviewed by Carol Sarlissian, MD. (May 27, 2022). Things that raise your chances of dementia.). [7]

- **Air Pollution:** Although we think of air pollution being a cause of lung problems, science is showing that the brain is directly impacted by air pollution. A health study covering ten years, 1996 – 2006, found that air pollution can cause not only inflammation and damage to the vascular system but also demonstrated that it can cause brain damage. (Bakalar, N. (June 22, 2015). Pollution may age the brain. The New York Times. http://well.blogs.nytimes.com/2015/06/22/pollution-may-age-the-brain/) [11]
- **Cardiovascular Factors:** A cardiovascular disease (CVD) is usually caused by plaque buildup in arteries around your heart (Atherosclerosis). That can slow blood flow to your brain and put you at risk for stroke, making it harder to think or remember things. And many things that cause heart disease – tobacco use, diabetes, high blood pressure, and high cholesterol – can lead to dementia.

    The main CVD risk factors that are known to increase a person's risk of getting dementia are:
1. High blood pressure
2. Increasingly stiff and blocked arteries (known as atherosclerosis)
3. High blood cholesterol levels
4. Being overweight and physically unfit
5. Type 2 diabetes (WebMD. Medically reviewed by Carol Sarlissian, MD. (May 27, 2022). Things that raise your chances of dementia.) [7]

Now before you breathe a sigh of relief and believe this synopsis was written for your parents or grandparents, or anyone older than you, let's look at how you accumulate risk factors throughout your life.

Here is an explanation of how we accumulate risk factors as we go through life:

The day we are born:

We have a clean slate – except if you were born with the **ApoE 4 gene.** Then you have started with a 7% risk of dementia.

Early Life:

Throughout your early life, you don't normally pick up any risk factors. If you have **less education** at this life stage, you pick up an 8% risk.

Midlife:

Midlife is the time that the body starts to pay for the wild and crazy life we might have been living. You increase your risk:

- 9% risk of **hearing loss**
- 2% risk with **hypertension**
- 1% risk with **obesity**

Late Life:

You pay the piper in late life and increase your risk with these poor lifestyle choices:

- 5% risk with **smoking**

- 4% risk with **depression**

- 3% risk with **physical inactivity**

- 2% risk with **social isolation**

- 2% risk with **diabetes**

All these risk factors add up to a **35% potentially modifiable risk.** These are all lifestyle issues that you can change if you choose to change.

Our Modifiable Risk Factors

Keith Fargo, Ph.D., director of scientific programs and outreach at the Alzheimer's Association states, "Research from the past two-three years suggests that risk factors need to be focused on in midlife." Dr. Douglas Scharre, a neurologist, advises that we should be addressing our modifiable risk factors no matter what our age is.

I have written about many of these risk factors over the years because I wanted to relate how they all play a factor in your chances of developing dementia. The increase in the number of risk factors you have does increase your potential of developing dementia. You have the choice and the means to change your life when you address the risk factors that you live with. Experts have focused on three different targets to reduce your risk of dementia: exercise, mental stimulation, and heart health. Get sweaty a few times a week but walking will provide some benefits too. Engage in as many activities that stimulate as many parts of the brain as possible. When you are having a conversation with other people you are stimulating large areas of your brain. Finally, a healthy heart will keep blood flowing to your brain, delivering needed oxygen and nutrients.

You can't change the genetics we were born with. But you do have the control to change the modifiable risk factors you take on throughout your life. It is estimated that 82 million people worldwide will have dementia by 2030. It is never too early or too late to change your brain. But you need to start now to ensure that you are not one of those 82 million people. Queensland Brain Institute. Dementia risk factors. https://qbi.uq.edu.au/dementia/dementia-risk-factors [12]

I didn't forget about stress. It is a powerful lifestyle factor that deserves a detailed section in the Lifestyle Plan in Chapter Eight.

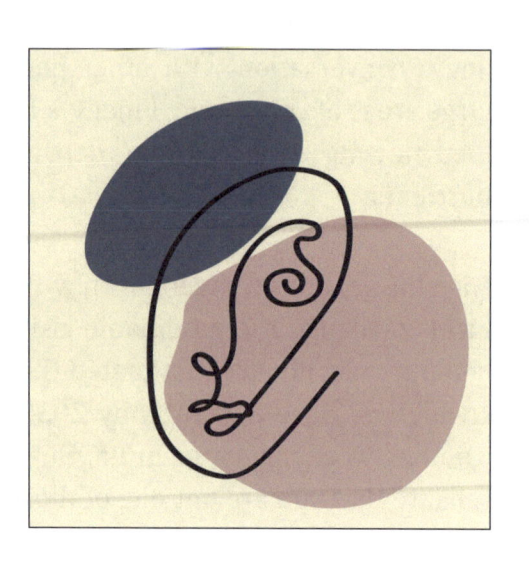

chapter eight

The PLAN for a Healthy Brain Lifestyle

In this chapter, you will find important information about the healthy brain lifestyle. There are six sections: Move/Physical Exercise, Challenge/Mental Stimulation, Nourish/Nutrition, Connect/Socialization, Sleep, and Calm/Stress.

Earlier in this book I reviewed risk factors associated with lifestyle and chronic disease. That might have seemed a bit daunting. This Plan explains how you can achieve a healthy brain by incorporating these lifestyle changes. This is all about changing your brain! Don't get overwhelmed by the lengthy content. There is no one lifestyle change you can make to recover your resilient brain. These six lifestyle components are synergistic; meaning, the whole is greater than the sum of the parts. Take each component and reflect on it. Each person is different and certain parts of each section will resonate individually. That will be your takeaway.

Chapter Eight will take this information and put it in a way that becomes your life plan without upending your life. Enjoy reading about the keys to longevity!

MOVE/PHYSICAL EXERCISE

A couple of years ago I broke two bones in my left foot. I was an avid walker and considered that my prime source of exercise. For 12 weeks I was on crutches and ordered to stay off my feet. That wrecked my exercise program. During that recovery time, I noticed that I was more fatigued and struggled to write my blogs. I was in a brain fog. My walking practice was severely interrupted, and I found it very hard to get back into the habit of walking. I knew how important it was, but my time off pushed me out of my groove. The moral is: Do your best to maintain your exercise practice, no matter what, for the sake of your brain.

Why Exercise?

Exercise works on the molecular and biochemical machinery of the brain. It helps create BDNF – brain-derived neurotrophic factor. BDNF acts as a fertilizer for new brain cells to bud from brain stem cells. With the help of BDNF, neurons maintain cell integrity and develop resistance to toxins and stress effects as they develop into mature neurons.

Our brains are hardwired for us to move our bodies. What does that even mean? We have inherited hardwiring — below our level of awareness — from our prehistoric ancestors. We were meant to move. Exercise is exceptionally good for our brain and brain function.

Physical exercise is one of the most researched elements of brain health. Technology has enabled researchers to see how the brain responds to exercise.

The brain needs nutrients to make energy. The prefrontal cortex is an energy cannibal. However, the brain is not a closed system where it has everything it needs to make energy. It needs to have nutrients sent to it. This little three-pound organ between our ears requires 20% of blood, carbohydrates, and oxygen from every heartbeat.

There is an intimate brain-heart connection. If you have a good heart, you will probably have a good brain, and vice versa. Exercise increases the blood flow to the brain. When you do any type of aerobic exercise, your heart beats faster and sends more nutrients to your brain. The nutrients stimulate the growth of new brain cells (neurons) and the connections between them.

How much exercise is necessary? Walking at a moderate pace of 30 minutes/day, 4-5x/week will help the brain. Dr. Cynthia Green, renowned for her continuing work on brain health, has created a Brain Power Walk – It goes like this: Get a partner to walk with you. This will hold you accountable. Start your walk at a pace where you can carry on a conversation. Walk at that pace for 10 minutes. Now bump your pace up so that it is too difficult to talk to each other. Again – walk this pace for 10 minutes. Then, for the last 10 minutes, scale back your pace to a conversational level. This will be your cool down. If walking isn't an option for you – you can try any type of aerobic exercise: swimming, bicycling, chair exercises, gardening, and dancing are excellent ways to get your aerobic exercise in.

Brain Benefits of Exercise

Research has shown that exercise improves brain function – the ability to be more creative, think clearer, and improve rational thinking. This makes sense when you think about it. All these functions are done in the prefrontal cortex. When you exercise you are getting your heart rate up and sending lots of nutrients to the prefrontal cortex so that it can function on a higher level. Think of this in terms of the workplace for a minute. You have a long meeting and not much gets accomplished, but you are completely drained of energy. That is because your prefrontal cortex used up all the energy it produced with the nutrients it had and drained out. The result is mental exhaustion. Now think about having a standing meeting where you are up and moving or better yet – a walking meeting. Your heart is beating faster and sending nutrients to your prefrontal cortex, and it functions at a high energy level — more ideas, more creativity, more everything.

Better mental health: research supports that depression and anxiety are reduced when you are physically active. And you are building brain resilience. I talked about building your brain at the beginning of this section. Brain resilience is the ability of the brain to function on a high level even if there is the presence of disease.

As you were getting older, you didn't notice the effect of cell or connection losses in your brain. This is because you had a lot of cells and connections to work with and if some were lost you wouldn't be able to notice a change. Now being a little older you don't have that same amount of cognitive reserve to work with anymore, and you can notice the losses. When we build more cognitive reserve by creating more cells and connections, we reduce the risk of cognitive decline and dementia.

This is what we are doing for our brain when we exercise and do all the other pieces of the healthy brain-for-life plan. We are making our brains strong again.

Health Consequences/Benefits of Exercise

Exercise decreases the risk of heart disease. Remember our heart is being pushed to function on a high level. This keeps our heart fit. The opposite side of the coin with this is if we don't exercise, we increase the risk and severity of cognitive decline and dementia. Remember – there is a direct connection between the brain and the heart. As an example, say you have congestive heart failure. With this disease, your heart doesn't beat strong enough to cause effective circulation. The brain would not get the nutrients it requires to function on a high level.

There is evidence that exercise can reduce the symptoms of depression and anxiety. Some studies indicate that exercise alone can lift depression. A note here — I will be telling you about many ways that a healthy lifestyle can alleviate chronic diseases, depression, and others. Please do not take it upon yourself to stop taking any medication because you heard or read something I said. I believe that this information is important and valuable, but you must talk with your doctor before you decide to stop taking any medication or go off your diet.

Right now, there is an obesity epidemic. Many chronic health conditions can accompany obesity. Cardiovascular disease, high blood pressure, and diabetes are all complications of obesity. Unfortunately, all these diseases put you at higher risk for dementia. A sedentary lifestyle is also part of the obesity puzzle. As I mentioned at the beginning of this section, our brains were made to move. Sitting in front of a computer or TV for six to eight hours each day puts us at a higher risk for dementia. It is a health concern that is receiving a lot of research attention. Being sedentary for six to eight hours/day is as dangerous as smoking 1- 1.5 packs of cigarettes a day. The Alzheimer's Assoc. made a statement that 1 in 7 cases of Alzheimer's could be prevented if those inactive took up exercise.

Exercise Effects on the Brain

Our brains produce neurotransmitters that serve a lot of different purposes. As we get older, production of these chemicals decreases. Exercise promotes a healthier output of these brain chemicals. Exercise lowers levels of inflammatory markers in the blood. Inflammation is your body's way of protecting itself from harmful stimuli including damaged cells, irritants, or pathogens. Infection is not the same as inflammation. Recent studies indicate that inflammation may be a primary cause of Alzheimer's disease. Exercise decreases the risk of heart disease (cardiovascular disease). Finally, it sparks the recovery process and leaves the body and mind stronger and more resilient to future stress.

Balance

I have a lot of experience with balance problems. As I mentioned in Chapter Five, I have Meniere's Disease a balance disorder that encompasses the inner ear, eyes, and brain. Over ten years, I've had three surgeries, stayed on a low-sodium diet, and fell numerous times. I was so sick with nausea from being so dizzy that I lost quite a bit of weight. It turned out that the right side of my brain was registering very little balance function. The vestibular system works by taking in visual and auditory signals and the brain keeps you balanced when those signals agree with each other. My right side had only a 15% balance function while my left side registered a 100% balance function. My brain could not justify the difference, so I had surgery. In 2012, I had vestibular nerve section surgery. This was one of those last-resort surgeries because I had tried everything else.

The otolaryngologist and the neurosurgeon did a craniotomy on the right side of my skull and clipped the vestibular nerve at the brain stem. The first post-op visit to the neurosurgeon was at three months. I was still a mess – I couldn't walk without a cane, and I still felt dizzy. Expressing my frustration with recovery to my doctor, I was met with this response, "At least you didn't come here in a wheelchair!" That answer stunned me. He then said it would take a year before I felt normal; meaning that there would be no dizziness. At my one-year visit, I still complained about dizziness and the response was, "It will probably be three years before the dizziness subsides." I was crushed by that news but the only thing I could do was to continue my balance rehab and get my brain back in order.

And just like that, it was around the three-year mark post-surgery that I felt I could walk straight and not feel like I would fall. My brain needed that much time for the power of neuroplasticity to make the left side of my brain take over the balance function of my whole brain! My brain did an amazing job with neuroplasticity.

Our balance system, the vestibular system, is composed of our eyes, our inner ear, and our brain. Input from the eyes and inner ear is transmitted to the brain where the brain compares the input and if both sides come in at 100% balance function, you continue to stand upright. What happens when the two sides of your brain don't agree? Most likely you will be experiencing dizziness or vertigo. The bigger the gap between the balance function of the two sides of the brain, the more incapacitated you are, and falling is likely to happen.

With all that said, our vestibular system does get weaker as we get older. But it is not an aging issue. It gets weaker because we do not challenge it. How can we do that? Let's start with something easy – if we take our daily walks on a walking trail or uneven surfaces, we are challenging our balance system. Our brain must make very small adjustments to make sure we stay upright. If you have some lower extremity weakness, use adaptive equipment, like a walker or a cane. They have some cool walking sticks on the market, and you can look hip!

Tai Chi is a moving meditation that is very slow deliberate movement. Tai Chi is excellent for balance training. There are balance rehab exercises you can do:

- Stand on one leg for at least 20 seconds then switch to

the other leg. I usually do this when I am waiting for the microwave to heat my food.

- Stand heel-toe and see if you can stand without losing your balance. Close your eyes while you are doing this. Many balance exercises can improve your vestibular system. There are balance centers where all the therapists evaluate you and determine what balance exercises would benefit you. Standing up without fear of falling is good.

Risk Factors for Falls

The first underlying risk is having a weakened vestibular system. If you have balance problems, get an evaluation. Having a fall can be deadly.

If you have had a previous fall, you are at risk for falling again. Meniere's disease is a balance disorder disease. Until the underlying issues of the disease are addressed you are at risk for multiple falls. Older adults can have Osteoporosis or Osteopenia and a fall can result in broken bones or necks.

- Physical limitations can put you at risk for falls. If you have lower extremity weakness or have had a stroke, or bad knees or hips — all of these, put you at risk of falling.
- More than one chronic condition can lead to falls. Chronic conditions include everything from diabetes, cardiovascular disease, arthritis, and COPD.
- Taking more than four medications can be a risk factor for falls. Our medications interact with each other. That can potentiate fall risk. Be alert to any signs of

dizziness. If it becomes difficult to walk because you are too dizzy, call your doctor. Multiple medications cause frequent falls.

- Anyone who is cognitively impaired is at risk for falls. Part of the disease process for a neurodegenerative disease is the inability to understand spatial relations. You can't figure out where you are in your own space. Taking a step forward is delicate — where are you stepping? Sitting down in a chair can be difficult — where is the chair to where you are standing?
- Lower body weakness and gait balance problems are the prime causes of falls. If you need hip or knee surgery or if you just had knee or hip surgery, rebuilding lower body strength is critical for mobility.
- Prolonged time in bed weakens lower extremities and moving from the bed to a chair becomes difficult.

Know your body. Get help if you need it. Falls are one of the leading causes of death among the older population.

CHALLENGE/MENTAL STIMULATION

My entry into the brain health field occurred around the year 2006. I was attending an American Society on Aging Conference and in the vendor area was a booth by Posit Science. They were introducing their Brain Fitness Program (BFP), and I was so awestruck by the fact that we could change our brains. It took a few years before I got to experience the BFP. This was more like neuro-rehab because the exercises were very tough. The BFP was an auditory processing program. The exercises improved the speed of processing, focus, and concentration, and helped with memory. It did make a big difference in my brain function. They then released Cortex with Insight, a visual processing program. There was more gaming in this program, and it was easier to complete. Now BFP is called BrainHQ and is one of the leaders in the field of online brain training. BrainHQ is an online subscription program from Posit Science. Check it out at http://www.brainhq.com. Online brain games are only one piece of mentally stimulating our brains. This section talks about many ways to challenge our brain and the benefits of neuroplasticity.

Our brain is always adapting to our environment – good or bad. You will learn how important our environment is in terms of a healthy brain.

Cognitive abilities define our state of brain function. I will cover the concept of cognitive reserve and how it impacts our aging brain.

Brain games are not the only way to challenge our brains and get results. You will learn about everyday practices that will keep your brain functioning at a high level.

And I will discuss memory. The fear of losing our memory is bigger than being diagnosed with cancer. We will review tools and strategies you can use to keep your memory sharp.

I include medications in this segment because they can wreak havoc on your memory. It can be so bad sometimes that you think you might be slipping into dementia. After we examine this, you will understand why.

Building Stronger Brains

You have started growing new brain cells through all your physical activity. Now you must use those cells. The brain is very good at pruning unused cells and connections. It is time to start challenging your brain!!

Our lifetime experiences, such as education and engaging in mentally challenging careers and activities, influence how our brains age. If we have been involved in novel and complex activities all our lives, our brain has benefitted by continually growing new neurons and new connections.

Our brain is constantly changing and adapting to our environment because of neurogenesis and neuroplasticity. Our brain changes for the good or the bad. If you are in a stimulating environment, your brain builds resilience. But if your environment is toxic, negative, or stress-ridden, your brain adapts to that also. Unfortunately, your brain ages quicker if you are in a negative environment. That means that you lose more cells and connections and brain function declines.

The conscious mental activities of cognition include the activities of thinking, understanding, learning, and remembering. These activities take place in the prefrontal cortex, the executive function center of the brain.

After the mid-twenties, our cognition starts to decline. We don't realize or feel that change because we usually have very healthy, vibrant brains that are full of cognitive reserve. Cognitive reserve is the massive number of neurons we accumulate through early brain development. These neurons offset the loss of brain volume as we grow older. Cognitive reserve provides the brain's resilience or ability to cope despite damage or degeneration. When we hit around the age of 50, we start to notice that we are forgetting things: What did I need at the store? What is that person's name? These memory lapses and tip-of-the-tongue phenomena can create a lot of angst. We can't see what is going on with our aging brain and so we might worry that we are on the slippery slope to dementia.

What has happened is that we have used our cognitive reserve over the years and now the losses of brain cells and connections are apparent in the troubles we are having with brain function.

We all vary in the amount of cognitive reserve we have. These differences are caused by genetics, education, occupation, lifestyle, leisure activities, and other life experiences. If we have constantly challenged ourselves to novel and complex activities, we are building cognitive reserve.

Now that we are older, we must work harder to rebuild this cognitive reserve to have a strong, healthy, high-functioning brain. The mental activity builds cognitive reserve. Only you can choose to challenge your brain and reap the benefits of a healthy, high-functioning brain. Your mental activities should be consistent, complex, challenging, and varied.

Different Ways to Challenge Your Brain

Here are some excellent activities that challenge your brain and help build brain reserve:

- **Lifelong Learning:** There are many programs available for seniors to be able to jump back into the learning arena: like the Osher Lifelong Learning Institute. OLLI is a national program usually run through local universities. I often lecture at OLLI operated through the University of Cincinnati.
- **Institute of Learning in Retirement ILR:** This is another program that is run through universities. I presented through the ILR program at Miami University in Oxford Ohio.
- **Travel:** There is little that can be more beneficial to the brain than travel. Everything is unique; languages might be different; you must navigate your way through the location you are visiting; and you are interacting with many different people. There is a huge brain benefit from travel.
- **Board games**: It is hard to imagine that board games can challenge your brain. However, if you think about it, many of them tap into your strategic skills, bring out the creative you, and sharpen your memory and reaction times.
- **Bridge:** There are so many strategy and memory skills involved with bridge. Plus, you are playing bridge with other people and socializing has a major impact on your brain.
- **Playing a musical instrument:** If you played an instrument when you were younger, pick it up and

start playing again. Or learn to play a new instrument. If you are a newbie at playing, there isn't a better time than the present. Learning how to read music and then playing an instrument has the broad benefits of learning a new language. Finger movements stimulate fine motor control. The perseverance and dedication to learning stimulate higher brain function.

- **Writing**: Again, there is not a better time to write. We are more creative as we get older. For one thing, we don't care if other people like what we create. Taking that barrier away can get the creative juices flowing.
- **Art:** Also, we are creative beings. Now we can let that creativity shine. The Alzheimer's Association has an art program, "Memories in the Making." This program is for individuals who have been diagnosed with Alzheimer's Disease and their artwork is amazing. Miami University in Oxford, Ohio, offers a program, "Opening Minds through Art "(OMA). This has resulted in beautiful art pieces and a higher quality of life for those diagnosed to be in the more advanced stages of Alzheimer's Disease.
- **Hobbies:** There are so many benefits of hobbies. When the hobby becomes very easy for you to do, you need to bump it up a notch. Your brain benefits from fumbling and learning in the beginning stages of a hobby.

Intelligence

Intelligence is the ability to reason, plan, solve problems, think abstractly, comprehend complex data, and learn quickly from experience.

There are two types of intelligence:

- **Fluid intelligence**: the ability to think logically, reason, and solve problems independent of education and knowledge. Fluid intelligence decreases with age.
- **Crystallized intelligence:** skills, knowledge, and experience learned during a lifetime – from family, at school, and from society. Crystallized intelligence increases with age. That is wisdom.

Online Brain training

I can't talk about mental stimulation without talking about online brain training. Many people believe that this is the only way to take care of their brain, or it is the fastest way to improve our brain. Online brain games do offer a lot of benefits. They are targeted to improve certain skills, such as concentration, focus, speed of processing, and reaction time.

The activities I mentioned at the beginning of this module challenge your whole brain. So far, the research has not supported the belief that these brain games can be generalized to better quality of life benefits. Can people think faster and remember more in real life because of playing these games or are they just better at the games themselves?

I believe the benefits of these games are going to continue to improve. But there is one clear thing – they must be a part of an entire healthy brain program. The brain is very complex, and these games won't take care of all the things we have to do to keep our brain healthy.

Here are a couple of the leaders in the field:

- Brain HQ by Posit Science
- Lumosity by Lumas Labs

There are many other online brain games. Before you get a subscription, make sure you like what the target functions are and the research that has been done to support their claims.

Go to https://brainhq.com to learn about Posit Science and its online games. There are a few you can try out and see if you like them.

Memory

One of the biggest scares as we get older is thinking that we are losing our memory. The normal aging issues of memory lapses can stop us cold, especially if you have had a family member who has had Alzheimer's disease. We are going to review memory and aging and put to rest some of the fear that pops up.

Semantic memory is the ability to recall concepts, numbers, words, and general facts that are not related to specific experiences. Let me give you an example: Understanding that a clock is used to tell time is obvious. Semantic memory also includes vocabulary and knowledge of language. Semantic memory continues to improve in aging.

Episodic memory: It captures what, where, and when of daily life. Think of this as episodes of a TV series. Episodic memory declines slightly as we age. An example of this is having trouble remembering what you went to the grocery store to get, or even having trouble remembering appointments.

Other brain functions that decline or slow down:

These include information processing and learning something new. I must use myself as an example of this. I went back to graduate school when I was 51 years old. All my classmates were around 25. When the professor asked a question of the group, they were already answering the question while I was trying to figure out what the question was! Luckily, we have amazing brains and I got mine up to speed as fast as I could.

Another function that declines is **cognitive flexibility.** This is known as mental multitasking. Let's say we have a couple of different streams of information coming into our brains. We want to compare or integrate the information to make a decision. Our aging brains don't work fast enough to be able to juggle all of this information and come up with a decision.

Dementia is not the only cause of memory problems even though it is the first thing everyone thinks about. It is important not to assume the worst. Get an evaluation from a geriatrician to determine the cause of memory problems. Other causes of memory problems can also be reversible, which is one of the primary reasons to get that evaluation. Anxiety, dehydration, depression, infections, medication side effects, poor nutrition, psychological abuse, and thyroid imbalance can also be blamed for memory problems. All these conditions are reversible. Don't live with fear — go get yourself checked out.

The big categories of memory function are short-term memory and long-term memory. It is important to understand how memory works to understand memory decline.

The first input signal of information destined to be memory comes into the prefrontal cortex (right behind the forehead). This signal is picked up by working memory. Working memory is vulnerable to distraction, it has limited storage capacity and only holds the information for a very short period. Seven to ten bits of information are the maximum amount that working memory can hold, for instance – a telephone number.

Working memory sends off the information to short-term memory and that makes its way to the hippocampus — the center of learning and memory. While you sleep at night, the hippocampus looks at the signals sent to it for embedding. If the signal was fuzzy, nothing happens. The signal wasn't strong enough to be embedded. If there is a clear signal, the hippocampus scans out and about the brain to find a similar memory and then consolidates the two. This makes the memory very strong, and it is more likely to be remembered, albeit a little different than the original memory itself. How can a signal be fuzzy? If we have untreated hearing loss – our brain can't interpret the signal coming in because it isn't clear. The same thing happens with vision problems. The signal must be clear and strong to make it a memory. While we are worried that we can't remember someone's name, the very likely possibility exists that we didn't make a memory in the first place. Remember, working memory is very vulnerable to distractions. We lose our filters for distractions as we get older, and it is harder to focus and pay attention. One of the strategies for making memories is to PAY ATTENTION and make a strong signal.

Long-term memory has unlimited capacity and is not vulnerable to distraction. Once the memory is embedded, it is there for good. If you don't recall the memory often, it loses its strength and may be harder and harder to recall.

These are some categories of long-term memory:

Implicit or Nondeclarative memory: this category includes habits and skills that we can do automatically, like driving a car.

Explicit or Declarative memory: these are memories we are consciously aware of and try to remember. There are two different kinds of explicit memory:

Episodic: memory of things; events that happened to you.

Semantic: more general knowledge.

Keep Your Memory Sharp

This book starts by stating something we never consider when we think our memory is declining: "Faltering memory may be a decline in the rate at which we learn and store new information."

So here are some suggestions to help you pay attention to the whole process and perhaps, increase your memory skills:

- **Relax**: Stress and tension are associated with memory lapses. Managing stress improves memory.
- **Concentrate:** Remember that our distraction filters aren't working very well anymore. Pay attention to remember.
- **Focus:** Seek to reduce distractions and interference. This is a skill that can be practiced.
- **Slow down**: Moving too fast? It is hard to focus and pay attention.
- **Organize:** Keep important and/or frequently used items in the same place, you don't have to think about where they are when you need them. You will create a habit by continually putting something in the same place repeatedly.
- **Write it down:** Give your brain a break. You aren't helping your brain when you try to remember everything. You are causing wear and tear – it is called cognitive load.
- **Repeat it:** Repetition improves recall. That is because you are adding strength to that signal, and it becomes easier to recall it.
- **Visualize it:** Our visual memory is very strong, but we don't use it to capacity. Creating a visual memory can help with recall.
- **Associate:** New information can be encoded strongly if it is associated with something that you already know or previously learned.

Staying Sharp: Memory and Aging: NRTA (AARP's Education Community and the Dana Alliance for Brain Initiatives.) [13]

Memory Aids

These are strategies for creating and remembering memories. These memory aides are very much like the memory strategies that were just reviewed in "Keep Your Memory Sharp." There are a couple of different applications to what was just learned, and let's go over those differences.

- **Keep "to-do" lists:** Lists are good; however, to-do lists can give you a feeling of accomplishment. When you complete a task, mark it off the list. It doesn't matter how simple or complex that task was. When you have crossed off all the tasks on your list – you will feel good and get a dose of dopamine released in your brain. Dopamine is the motivating reward neurotransmitter. Production of that slows down as we get older, so anytime we can stimulate production – we are helping our brain.
- **Establish a routine:** When we do this, we are creating habits that are run by our subconscious brain. We don't have to consciously think about what we are doing. Your brain is automatically directing us to do it, and we don't forget as much.
- **Don't rush:** Again, our brains are running a little slower. We need more time to remember a name or recall a new one. Give yourself a break by not putting so much pressure on your brain.
- **Everything in its place:** We talked about this earlier. If you consistently put things in the same place, you

don't have to think about where they are. It reduces stress too.

- **Use associations:** Whenever we can give our brain a cue to help with recall, we are far more successful in remembering. Associations are a strong tool for memory. I will use my last name as a memory association tool. Faust is my last name. There is a famous opera titled FAUST. If you are aware of the opera, when you hear my name, you will form an association with that title and never forget my name!

- **Tag new information:** This is a memory technique to help with recall. This takes some practice, but if you take the time to perfect this technique, you may never need a list again. Here is an example: You have five things you need to get at the hardware store. Have a room design from your house in mind. Say you use the family room: a shiny new hammer on top of the TV; a roll of duct tape on the seat of your favorite chair and so on. Use the same furniture layout for everything and just replace the items you need to remember. It takes a little practice, but this is an old strategy with success.

- **Keep a calendar:** Doesn't matter what kind of calendar you use – write all appointments, events, birthdays, anniversaries, etc. in your calendar. Then you won't have to worry about forgetting anything. If you get a universal calendar. It has just months and dates – no years. You can put your information in one time and use it year after year! It is a huge relief to set this memory tool up. (American Psychological Association) [14]

Medications and Aging

We are going to take another sidestep to look at medications. I include this segment in "Challenge" because medications can wreak havoc with your memory. It can be so bad sometimes that you think you might be slipping into dementia. After we examine this, you will understand why.

Even though we don't have a lot of research to support how our older bodies react and process medications, the dilemma persists. We might have taken a certain medication for several years. There were never any significant side effects. Now, over the past few months, you find that you just aren't feeling that good anymore. Nothing has changed, except your aging body. You are also taking maybe five or six medications, perhaps each one being added on to deal with new chronic conditions. As the meds keep adding up, it is hard to tell how they are interacting with each other. Should you find difficulties in taking all these medications, you can go straight to the doctor and ask for a medication evaluation or go to your pharmacist and ask for some advice. That is their job. Or they could recommend that you see your ordering physician.

Our brain ages as we get older. It is changing shape and function. Everything starts with the brain and these aging changes might interfere with medication metabolism. You could have unexpected side effects because of your changing, aging brain.

We have already mentioned that as we get older, our metabolism slows down. This is an important fact to know when you start thinking of taking your medications. There isn't enough good information available to specifically tell us how fast we metabolize and then clear medications. All research studies are done on younger, healthy individuals. We can take our medicine and it might not be cleared by the time we take our next dose. A residual effect can occur when we are building up the levels of medicine in our bodies, and this can be a problem.

In addition, your circulatory and digestive systems as well as your liver and kidneys all slow down and can affect how fast medicines enter and leave your body. So, we have slowing metabolism and slowing organs interacting with processing medications.

Weight changes can play a significant role in how much medicine you need and how long it stays in your body. Perhaps you have gained weight, and your dosages aren't high enough to make a difference in your actions. Perhaps you got sick, and you lost significant weight. Your medications may now be too strong for your body weight. It is important to talk with your doctor if this happens to you.

Multiple medications can interact with each other as well as, food, drink, vitamins, supplements, natural products, alcohol, and/or other existing health problems. It is good to have a pharmacist as your gatekeeper when you are taking multiple medications.

One thing that slips by in the analysis is the over-the-counter drugs (OTC). OTCs are still potent drugs. Just because we don't need to have a prescription doesn't diminish their potency. Aspirin, for example, is an anticoagulant, meaning it thins your blood. In combination with other drugs, it can cause you to bleed. If you are already on an anticoagulant, you do not want to take aspirin. Supplements and vitamins can interact and interfere with your medications. That is why you need to establish a relationship with a pharmacy/pharmacist.

Medications, Aging, and Cognitive Function

Cognition is a person's ability to think, understand, learn, plan, and remember. Cognitive decline starts in our mid-twenties. Medications can play havoc with your brain at any age, but you are more vulnerable to problems when you are older. Some side effects of medications can cause serious health problems which include effects on a person's cognition.

Side effects that target brain function include:

- Problems concentrating or paying attention
- Confusion
- Memory loss
- Hallucinations or delusions

This is no laughing matter. Through my years in the healthcare system, I have seen several people who have been treated for dementia, when really, they were over-medicated or medicated with the wrong drugs. There have even been some cases where an individual has died because they didn't look at medications as a cause of health or cognitive problems. I want to take this moment to ask you to advocate for someone older if they are caught in the healthcare system. And designate someone to look out for you as you get older. If an individual is exhibiting any of the above-mentioned conditions, get a geriatric evaluation. Geriatricians are specialists in diagnosing and treating older adults. They view the older body in a very different way.

NOURISH / NUTRITION

The brain is very picky about its nutrients. When you start to think about all the activities the brain is involved in, you begin to understand how the food you eat is so important to brain function. The brain is the center of everything, and it requires a lot of different nutrients for energy and function.

The nutrition information is a bit heavy on the science side. I don't want you to get bogged down with all the science. You must have a simple working memory of what the brain requires so that you make smart choices in what you eat. Currently, nutrition is undergoing a huge leap forward in understanding what the brain needs. The Brain-Gut connection is one of the hottest research topics right now, and the research is bearing out a lot of big discoveries.

There is a lot to learn. So, let's get started.

What Does the Brain Need to Function?

As they say, "You are what you eat!" The foods we eat or don't eat impact our brain, mental health, and mood. That is a lot to comprehend. How can one aspect of our lives mean so much and make such an impact?

Our brain is very specific in its needs. It needs Oxygen, Carbohydrates, and Blood. Our brain is the fattiest organ in our body; it is 60% fat. So, we need to send good fat to it also. High protein foods help balance blood sugar and ensure a steady supply to our brain.

Here is a list of required dietary needs for our brain for it to function on a high level:

1. **Fatty Acids**: As I just mentioned – our brain is 2/3 fat, and it requires a steady stream of fatty acids to keep cell membranes intact and insulate nerves. Omega-3 fatty acids are the best fats for the brain. A diet high in these fats helps prevent neurodegenerative diseases, like Parkinson's and Alzheimer's.

2. **Antioxidants**: Vitamins C and E protect delicate brain structures from free-radical damage, particularly to the fats that insulate nerve cells. Free radicals are atoms, or groups of atoms with an odd (unpaired number of electrons), and can be formed when oxygen interacts with certain molecules. Once free radicals form, the brain is especially vulnerable to free radical attacks. Antioxidants bind with those rogue oxygen molecules so that they won't do more damage. That is why you see so many food products labeled as antioxidants. They are very important to brain health.

3. **B-Complex Vitamins**: These vitamins keep your brain healthy by reducing the level of homocysteine, a byproduct of protein metabolism that promotes inflammation in the brain and the body. Excess homocysteine can cause inflammation within the blood vessel wall, which can decrease blood supply to

the brain. It can also directly damage brain cells that control coordination and reaction speed.

4. **Protein**: High-protein foods help to balance blood sugar and ensure a steady supply of glucose to the brain. Tyrosine, an amino acid in protein foods, such as meat, fish, and tofu, is a precursor needed to make neurotransmitters, dopamine, and norepinephrine. These are brain chemicals that affect your moods and energy levels. L-tryptophan, in poultry, milk, and eggs is a precursor of serotonin, a calming neurotransmitter that boosts mood and energy levels.

5. **Glutamine,** found in protein-rich foods, contributes to the production of gamma-aminobutyric acid, or GABA, an important neurotransmitter for reducing anxiety.

What Is the Best Diet for Your Brain?

We just covered all the essential components of the food we eat that affect the brain in many ways including wellbeing and mental health. There are bad mood foods. These are highly processed snacks and takeout food products rich in sugar and fats. I know that I just told you that our brain needs sugar and fats, but it needs the right kind of these nutrients.

There is a diet that fits all the criteria required for our brain to function properly. This diet has been widely researched over the past few years and is recognized as being just right for a healthy brain.

The MIND DIET is a combination of the Mediterranean diet and the DASH diet. The Alzheimer's Association has given strong support to the MIND diet. The MIND Diet List was put together by the Alzheimer's Association. It gives you the breakdown of foods you should eat and how many times per week you should eat them. You can keep track of your week's dietary intake and see how you do. One of the activities I am suggesting is to keep a journal of what you are eating. Having the truth in front of you speaks volumes.

The MIND Diet List (Alzheimer's Association)

- Green Leafy Vegetables: 6+ servings/week
- Other Vegetables: 7+ servings/week
- Berries 2+ servings/week
- Nuts 5+ servings/week
- Olive Oil Primary oil used
- Butter, Cream <1 serving/day
- Regular Cheese <1 serving /week
- Whole Grains 3+ servings/day
- Fish (not fried; not shelled) 2+meals/week
- Beans >3 meals/week
- Poultry (not fried) 2+meals/week
- Red Meat <3 meals/week

Some of the components of the MIND Diet are:

- Lots of plants - especially dark leafy vegetables and dark-skinned fruits
- Legumes, beans, and whole grains are included in this category
- Lots of healthy fat from cold water fatty fish such as mackerel, salmon, sardines, nuts, and olive oil
- Low in red meat and dairy.

Since the Mediterranean diet is a large part of this diet, you can refer to books on the Mediterranean diet to help guide you. Whole food diets protect against Alzheimer's disease, slow aging, and help prevent depression and anxiety.

Food and Dementia

I referred to "what's good for the brain is good for the heart" in the first module. This is basic nutrition. The two most common types of dementia affecting older adults, Alzheimer's disease, and vascular dementia, might be delayed by the same types of food and diets that help lower blood pressure, reduce cholesterol, and prevent or manage diabetes.

It is critical to lower our intake of bad fats (saturated and unsaturated fats). This has been in the news for quite a few years. Remember when the uproar was about all the fast food being fried in trans-saturated fat? It was a very big deal when the big fast-food places stopped doing that. (We need to cut our fast-food intake anyway.)

Heart health is all about cutting your cholesterol levels. With that said, if you increase more whole plant foods in your diet – that is better. The body adjusts and adapts to food intake and reacts much better. Whole plant foods pull cholesterol out of the body and flush it away. Fruits, vegetables, beans, whole grains, peas, and lentils make up the whole plant food group.

Berries, especially dark-skinned berries like blueberries, not only fight free radicals, but they also combat cholesterol, because they have a lot of soluble fiber.

You must increase your intake of monosaturated fats. Remember, your brain needs good fats, like omega-3 fatty acids. Your body does much better on food sources rather than supplements. There is some controversy over omega-3 fatty acid supplements or fish oil supplements. Studies have found that the supplement hasn't been a huge benefit for the brain. If you are eating a good variety of foods, you will be getting your needed antioxidants and vitamins. If you need to take a vitamin or a supplement, it is suggested that you take these at lunch because your metabolism is charged up and you can absorb the ingredients more effectively. Also, get liquid vitamins. Then you don't have to break down the components to metabolize them. You can find these in various places, and they are especially good for kids.

Again, your goal should be a diet with a higher intake of vegetables and fruit. If you look at your Mind Diet List, you will see that you should have six servings of green leafy vegetables a week. Also, recommended, that other vegetables should be eaten seven servings a week and berries should be eaten at least two servings per week.

The Do's and Don'ts of Nutrition

First, we must say no to so much red meat. We should have lots more vegetables on our plates. If you do eat red meat, make sure it is a lean cut of meat. Our brains and our hearts benefit from cutting back on meat.

The brain needs lots of green leafy vegetables and dark-skinned fruits. I know I am repeating myself with this, but this should give you some idea of how important this is. Dark-skinned fruit is chock full of antioxidants. The natural blue and purple pigments in berries can cross the brain-blood barrier. The brain-blood barrier is a protective mechanism for the brain. It is one of the reasons that vitamins and supplements might not work. Their components might not make it through the blood-brain barrier, and they don't do anything. Food sources break down and can get through that brain-blood barrier.

There is a fish tale when it comes to brain health. Cold water fatty fish (salmon, mackerel, tuna) are some examples. Baked or grilled, fish should become your next favorite food!!

Dark Chocolate!! Woohoo! Dark chocolate is full of flavonoids, which have serious antioxidants that protect your brain. The cocoa content should be high, and the quality of the chocolate should be good. If the cocoa content isn't high enough, then there is the possibility that increased bad fat exists. If you don't like the taste of high cocoa content – keep giving it a try. You will get used to it, and it becomes quite a treat. Finally, do not diet! It is healthier and better to follow these guidelines.

This Is Your Brain On:

Let's start with **Sugar**.

Too much sugar is linked to weight gain, obesity, type 2 diabetes, and heart disease. Wow! Sugar packs a big punch. Most times, we don't even realize how much sugar we take in during the day. It is hidden in processed foods, and fast foods and blatantly open in candy, snacks, ice cream, cookies, and all the other good stuff we know is bad for us. Sugar stimulates dopamine production, the feel-good neurotransmitter. What happens when you fight with your significant other, or the kids have pushed you over the top, or work is a catastrophe? You go eat sugar. It makes you feel good, but it is like anything else, too much is not good for you.

Diabetes: a high risk factor for cognitive decline and dementia.

Grains and Gluten: Refined grains are linked to obesity and many metabolic diseases, which are correlated with dementia. Whole grains tend to be high in fiber and various important nutrients. They do not have the same metabolic effects as refined grains. Evidence for gluten-causing dementia in people who do not have gluten sensitivity is weak and over-hyped. You need to reduce refined grains, like white rice, and white flour, but include whole grains in your diet.

Coffee: It is high in antioxidants (yay), and two to three cups a day is associated with a decreased risk of developing dementia.

Alcohol: Low to Moderate alcohol use is associated with a reduced risk of developing dementia. This statement is still being debated by science. Whereas one to two drinks a day was considered beneficial, science is pointing to zero alcohol consumption as being the healthiest option for the brain and body.

Omega-3s: What more can I say? Eating cold-water fatty fish is best!!

Ultra-processed Food: AACK!!!

Why the big AACK!! Do you ask? Ultra-processed food is junk food — the food we love and are addicted to. These are your microwavable dinners, deli meat, white bread, packaged cookies, cheese puffs, pastries, and fast food. They make up most of the packaged foods you find in the frozen food aisle, and on the menu of fast-food restaurants.

"Ultra-processed foods are formulated to be so palatable and satisfying that they are almost addictive," said Dr. Eric M. Hecht, an epidemiologist at the Schmidt College of Medicine at Florida Atlantic University. "The problem is that to make the products taste better and better, manufacturers make them taste less and less like real food." (Sally Wadyka, May 4, 2023, The New York Times). [15]

I like ultra-processed foods. They are convenient and tasty! But they are so bad for your health and your brain.

The Gut-Brain Microbiome Connection

The microbiome is 100 trillion bacterial cells that reside in your digestive tract. A healthy balance of gut microbes contributes to normal behavior, cognition, emotional regulation, and a well-functioning immune system. The human microbiome impacts physical, mental, and emotional health. The health of the gut and the health of the mental/emotional body are linked.

Your microbiome communicates with your enteric nervous system (the second brain of nerve tissue in your gut), your autonomic nervous system (your fight or flight and rest and digest branches of your nervous system), and your central nervous system (the brain and spinal cord). The chain of communication goes both ways — giving and receiving input.

Disruptions in gut-brain signaling may lead to abnormal brain function, changes in behavior, thoughts, emotions, and perceptions of pain, and may also impact our immune system. There is some support for a role in probiotics, but clinical evidence is still limited. Your gut flora, your bacteria, spurs serotonin production and signaling. Serotonin is not the only hormone involved when it comes to depression.

I found this part especially interesting. The gastrointestinal system has a large role in serotonin synthesis, use, and cycling. Ninety percent of serotonin creation occurs in the digestive tract, which also houses the largest number of serotonin receptors — way more than the brain!

Alcohol – the Rules Have Changed

I have found over the years that talking or writing anything about alcohol is looked at with a different perspective. No one wants to know what alcohol can do to your brain. It has planted itself in the fabric of our culture.

Benefits and Risks of Drinking Alcohol

Let's look at the risks first. Remember that we have aging bodies, and the metabolism of aging bodies slows down. Besides our metabolism, our organs involved in clearing have slowed down too. Specifically, our liver – the liver is known as the detoxifying organ. Wear and tear, overuse, and aging itself can slow liver processing.

Because the aging process affects how the body handles alcohol, the same amount of alcohol can have a greater effect as the person gets older. This can get us into trouble. We don't notice or pay attention to changes that might be occurring, so we see no problem in having our cocktails, beers, or wine at the same pace we always did. With this lack of insight, over time, someone whose drinking habits haven't changed may find he or she might have a serious drinking problem.

Now there have been some studies of this: Researchers found more brain tissue loss in those with alcoholism than in those without, and age renders a person more susceptible to alcohol.

- The frontal lobes are more susceptible and that is associated with intellectual impairment.
- Age-related changes in the volume of the brain also occur in the cerebellum, which is associated with stability; and regulates posture and balance.
- This, in turn, increases the likelihood of falls.

Alcohol does have some benefits for the body. The main reason a drink may be beneficial is because it is good for the heart and blood vessels. Alcohol thins the blood and reduces clotting. It also boosts good cholesterol. There is no strong scientific consensus that alcohol benefits the brain.

CONNECT/SOCIALIZATION

Social connection is paramount to health and wellness. We are hardwired to connect. In this section, we will look at how important it is to be with other people. We build cognitive reserve when we socialize, and this benefit reduces your risk of developing dementia.

We also need to connect within ourselves — to find that reason to get up in the morning. People who have passion and purpose in their lives have reduced their dementia risk.

Socialization is one of the primary drivers of brain health. I think you will like what you are going to hear. I love this section.

The Need to Connect

Social interaction is the key to cognitive development and function from a young age. However, staying socially active is very important for our brain, as it staves off and slows down the mental decline associated with dementia. Much of the chronic diseases and brain health or illness are a result of biological, psychological, and social factors.

"Socializing doesn't just help prevent mental disease, it can also help us to remember more and think more clearly. Oscar Ybarra of the University of Michigan, monitored phone usage data from 3600 people, analyzing how long they talked and to whom. Even while controlling for other variables, researchers uncovered a positive relationship between social engagement and cognitive performance."

(http://psp.sagepub.com/cgi/reprint/34/2/248)

We are hardwired to connect. It was a survival mechanism for our prehistoric ancestors. Being together – kept them alive. We still have the same need for social connection. By definition – social connection is the perception and reality that you are cared for, have assistance available from other people, and are part of a supportive social network. These supportive resources can be emotional, tangible (money), informational, or companion.

Measures of Social Connection

These are measures of social connection:

- Whether someone is married or not
- Lives with other people
- Has minimal monthly contact (including face-to-face, telephone, or written/e-mail contact) with children, or other family members or friends
- And, if they participate in social clubs, resident's groups, religious groups, or committees

Neuroscience research shows that being socially connected protects the brain against the risk of developing dementia and improves health and well-being.

- Women from large social networks (note: this study didn't include Facebook friends) have a lower risk of cognitive decline.
- Loneliness is associated with more than double the risk of developing dementia.

The Power of Socialization

How Friends and Family Impact Cognitive Reserve

People with stronger social relationships have an increased likelihood of survival than those with weaker social relationships.

Three of the nine "Blue Zones centenarians" behaviors involve social connection: belonging to a faith community, putting loved ones first, and belonging to the right tribe. Blue Zones are locations around the world where people live to very extended ages with strong physical and cognitive capabilities. Loma Linda is a location in the United States designated as a Blue Zone. Residents are members of the Seventh Day Adventists. They look out for each other, socialize together, eat healthy, and are very active. One gentleman that was featured as a member of this group, was a physician. At 97 he not only continued to do a full schedule of surgery, he was also able to cut his grass and do other activities that are usually associated with a much younger person.

Just because people with healthy brains tend to socialize more often, we can't say that socializing leads to brain health; but it's a contributor.

A research study looked at this correlation. Participants were assigned to one of three groups: a "social" group that participated in group discussion, an "intellectual activities" group that solved puzzles, and a control group that watched television. The groups met three times a week for ten weeks. They were given cognitive tests before the start of the study and then again upon completion of the study. Results: Those who spent their time socializing scored the highest — even better than the intellectual activities group!

The Fundamental Need to Connect

Participating in many different leisure activities builds brain resilience. Social interaction involves many cognitive functions, such as thinking, feeling, sensing, reasoning, and intuition.

Research shows these are the main benefits of having an active social life:

- You may live longer: People with more social support tend to live longer than those who are more isolated, and this is true even after accounting for your overall health.
- You will enjoy better physical health: Social engagement is associated with a stronger immune system, especially for older adults.

- This means that you are better able to fight off colds, the flu, and even some types of cancer.
- You will enjoy better mental health: Interacting with others boosts feelings of well-being and decreases feelings of depression. Research has shown that one sure way of improving your mood is to work on building social connections.
- You may even lower your risk for dementia. People who connect with others generally perform better on tests of memory and other cognitive skills. In the long run, people with active social lives are less likely to develop dementia than those who are more socially isolated.

These mentally stimulating activities build up our reserve of healthy brain cells and promote the formation of new connections, or synapses, between neurons.

Social Anxiety and Pain

The pregenual anterior cingulate cortex (pACC) is a key brain area involved in physical pain and social pain, which is responsible for processing unpleasant emotions caused by physical pain and negative emotions caused by social events.

Experiences of social rejection, exclusion, or loss are generally considered to be some of the most "painful" experiences that we endure. Negative social experiences have a profound effect on our emotional well-being.

The neural circuitry underlying physical and social pain overlaps. Physical and social pain rely on shared neural substrates. Factors that influence physical pain also alter social pain, like pain relievers, opiates, and social support.

So, what does all that mean?

Researchers used functional MRI (fMRI) to monitor the brain activity of study participants. A video depicting a person falling and hurting themselves was shown to a study participant under fMRI imaging. Researchers were able to note what part of the brain experienced this pain.

Then the same participants were shown a video of a person being humiliated by their boss in front of co-workers. The very same part of the brain showed activity to this social pain. There is one other interesting point about this. The effects of social pain never go away. If the incident is triggered the brain will perceive this pain repeatedly. Whereas physical pain does go away, emotional pain stays with you. Taking a pain reliever like acetaminophen or ibuprofen will relieve social pain.

Passion, Purpose, and Brain Health

When you retire your life changes. Whether you are prepared for these changes or not will determine how you will live your remaining years. Instead of being energized and inspired by the years ahead, you may be drained and lethargic. You are missing purpose. We search for what makes us happy at each stage of our journey. But we often spend more time planning our vacations than planning our lives. This is where purpose comes in: it is a combination of your skills, passions, and values.

"When you live a life you love, with people you love, doing the work that you love, you add years to your life and life to your years." Richard Leider, life coach.

(http://www.aarp.org/personal-growth-/transitions/info-06-2011/5-weeks-ep5-purpose.html) [16]

People who have meaning and purpose in their lives lower their risk of cognitive decline, mental health issues, and dementia. Why is that? They are immersed in their purpose and passion and are making their brains stronger and more resilient. Purpose in life is linked to positive health outcomes including better mental health, less depression, more happiness, satisfaction, self-acceptance, better sleep, and longevity.

1. **Live Longer:** Dan Buettner (researcher of Blue Zones) identified the factors that most centenarians share and one of them is a strong sense of purpose. In 2014, researchers used data that tracked adults over 14 years and found that "having a purpose in life appears to widely buffer against mortality risk across the adult years."

2. **Protect against heart disease:** Purpose is a possible protective factor against near-future myocardial infarction among those with coronary heart disease.

3. **Prevent Alzheimer's disease:** In a study of thousands of older subjects, Dr. Patricia Boyle, a neuropsychologist at the Rush Alzheimer's Disease Center in Chicago, found that people with a low sense of purpose were 2.4 times more likely to get Alzheimer's disease than those with strong purpose. Further, people with

purpose were less likely to develop impairments in daily living and mobility disabilities.
4. **Handle pain better:** Purpose can also positively affect pain management.

Purpose

I have already introduced the concept of purpose, but let's see what it is defined as. Purpose is the psychological tendency to derive meaning from life's experiences and to possess a sense of intentionality and goal-directedness that guides behavior.

What does that mean you might be thinking? Our brain likes a little structure. It functions better when clear goals are established. You turn your thoughts and actions to accomplishing those goals. Intentionality just means that you're fully immersed in that goal and attention and intention are focused on it.

One of the common features among people who live with purpose is that they find meaning in the things that happen to them. Andrew Zolli, the author of *Resilience,* describes these people as being able to "cognitively reappraise situations and regulate emotions, turning life's proverbial lemons into lemonade."

More research suggests that people with a strong sense of purpose are better able to handle the ups and downs of life. Purpose can offer a psychological buffer against obstacles. So, a person with a strong sense of purpose remains satisfied with life even when experiencing a difficult day. According to Barbara Fredrickson, this kind of long-term resilience can lead to better cardiovascular health, less worry, and greater happiness over time.[17]

Hunting for purpose:

Here are a few lists of things you can do to find your purpose. There is an agreement among experts in this field that there are some preliminary questions you should ask yourself as you start this process:

- Think about everything you have done in your life, beginning with your first jobs in your teen years. Then ask yourself these questions:
- What have I done that didn't seem like work?
- What have I done that I've never grown tired of doing?
- What have I done that energized me, either intellectually or emotionally?

The answer to these questions will lead you to your passion.

Here is a different perspective to elaborate on finding purpose:

1. **Don't let yourself rust out.** That is coach Richard Leider's term for what happens when we are gridlocked by life's circumstances and don't know how to break free.

"If you are spending precious hours feeling half-alive, dragging yourself through tasks you abhor, you're rusting out. Whenever you are not challenged by your life, whenever you feel like you're just going through the motions, it's time to rethink your purpose."

2. **Push the pause button:** What would be one thing you would change in your life if you could? People often respond to that question by expressing that they wished they had been more reflective. Too often we allow the busyness of our lives to hijack our sense of purpose. We are so caught up in doing what we must do, we lose track of what we want to do.

3. **Define your passion:** What's missing in your life? What are you curious about? What issues or problems do you feel strongly about?

"Think about what gets you up in the morning and keeps you up at night," says Leider. "I am not talking about worries and anxieties, but rather the interests and activities that excite and motivate you, or the causes you'd like to know more about and participate in."

Make a list of things you enjoy doing and believe you do well.

4. **Draw your life map:** This will help you visualize what you want and why you want it. Cut out pictures from magazines or download online images that calm you, inspire you, spur you into action, make you happy, and represent your life goals and dreams.

5. **Identify your brain trust:** Going it alone, without input from others, can keep you stuck. Ideally, you should have one person in your life you can count on just to listen when you need to work out options in your mind. You need another person to act as a catalyst, spurring you to act. And you need a wise elder — ten years your senior who can serve as a mentor and provide perspectives.

6. **Take it in stages:** Putting purpose into action demands motivation, courage, and patience. Start small. "Purpose evolves as interests and experiences change, and as you go through different ages and stages."

7. **Finally – write a personal mission statement to guide you on this journey.** [18]

Meaning

Meaning in our life comes from seeing a cause bigger than ourselves. It could be a specific deity or religion, or a cause that helps humanity in some way. The people coming to help and assist victims of hurricanes must find meaning in what they are doing.

We all need meaning in our lives to have a sense of well-being.

In defining purpose in life, Dr. Patricia Boyle states: **It's the sense that your life has meaning. You are engaged in things that energize and motivate you, and that you think are important on a broader level, beyond just yourself.** [19]

The more we feel engaged in life, the happier we are. But once we feel cut off from the flow and interaction of life, we are more likely to wither in body and mind.

SLEEP

Who doesn't want to talk about sleep? Right? Sleep is very important for a healthy brain.

We are going to examine the magic that happens in our brains while we are sleeping. Our brains have a cleaning system I will talk about, and we make our memories while we sleep.

Get ready to appreciate sleep on a whole other level!

What Is Sleep?

Why do we spend one-third of our life asleep? An obvious answer might be that we recover from the fatigue of being awake, to be ready for another day of challenges, good or bad.

We all know how it feels to not sleep: everything requires extra effort; we lack energy and motivation and feel groggy, irritable, and snappish. Sleep is not a period of rest, however. Our brain is very busy during sleep and serves an active, essential function.

Sleep loss or chronic sleep disruption has many negative consequences, including adverse effects on metabolism and immune function. The most obvious of these adverse effects are on the brain. Cognitive deficits of many kinds are apparent after just one night of total sleep deprivation or when sleep is cut short by several hours every night for a week or more.

Attention, working memory, and the ability to learn and remember decline. When we are sleep-deprived, it is more difficult to speak fluently, assess risks, and appreciate humor. More importantly, experiments have shown that these cognitive impairments can be reversed but not by the same period of "quiet wakefulness." There is evidence that cognitive deficits caused by sleep loss at night can be prevented or delayed by naps.

Sleep versus Rest

What distinguishes sleep from quiet, restful wakefulness? Sensory disconnection is the answer. During quiet restfulness, when we sit on a sofa in a silent dark room after having exercised, our muscles can recover from fatigue. Yet, we are still able to react and move promptly if the phone rings. We are still connected to the world. On the other hand, when deeply asleep, our capacity to react to a mild stimulus a noise coming from the next room, or that phone call — is reduced substantially. So, we must consider that when asleep, we are essentially offline: sensory disconnection must be an essential requirement for whatever function sleep serves. There are two types of sleep:
- **REM** – rapid eye movement and **NREM** – non-rapid eye movement
- **NREM sleep** can be broken down into three distinct stages: N1, N2, and N3. In the progression from stage N1 to N3, brain waves become slower and more synchronized. Stage N3 is referred to as "deep" or "slow wave" sleep.

- **REM sleep** is characterized by low amplitude, high-frequency waves and alpha rhythms, and eye movement. When people wake from REM sleep, they often report vivid, and sometimes bizarre dreams.
- Time spent each day awake, in REM sleep, and NREM sleep changes over a lifetime.

Circadian Rhythms

Your circadian rhythm (also known as your sleep/awake body clock) is a natural, internal system that's designed to regulate feelings of sleepiness and wakefulness over 24 hours. This complex timekeeper is controlled by an area of the brain that responds to light, which is why humans are most alert while the sun is shining and are ready to sleep when it is dark out.

Your circadian rhythm causes your level of wakefulness to rise and dip throughout the day. Most people feel the strongest desire to sleep between 1 pm to 3 pm and then again between 2 am and 4 am – but this can vary from person to person.

Your circadian rhythm can also change as you age. If you follow your natural cues regarding when you go to sleep and wake up, your circadian rhythm should stay balanced, but a change in your schedule can disrupt your body clock.

Follow these four tips to keep your circadian rhythm functioning as it should:

1. **Stick to a Consistent Sleep Schedule**. A regular bedtime is one part of the equation, but waking up at the same time daily will also help keep your circadian rhythm in check. It may be tempting to grab some

extra sleep on weekends, but doing so can throw off your body clock during the week.

2. **Go for an A.M. Walk.** In the morning, exposure to the sun (or indoor light) won't just give you an energy boost, it can also reset your circadian rhythm. A quick outdoor stroll in the morning will give you enough sun exposure to signal to your brain that it is time to start the day. No time to walk? Simply raise the blinds or switch on your brightest light instead.

3. **Go for a P.M. Walk.** To unwind after a busy day, take an evening walk. Walking with a friend in those evening hours can be very relaxing. Be mindful that this is the time to relax. Enjoy the sunset.

4. **Limit Evening Tech.** Bright lights in the evening hours can throw off your body clock by confusing your brain into thinking it is still daytime. Artificial blue light (the types that laptops, tablets, and cell phones emit) is the worst culprit; so, try to power down tech devices at least two to three hours before bed.

Why Do We Sleep?

Sleep was originally believed to keep us safe at night, conserve energy, and allow our bodies to rest and repair. But as research dug into our brain function while we sleep it uncovered a long list of brain functions that occur. Our brain is almost as busy while we are sleeping as when we are awake.

Let's take a look:

- **Clear out toxins:** Dr. Maiken Nedergaard of the University of Rochester Medical Center along with her colleagues, discovered a system that drains waste products from the brain. Cerebrospinal fluid (CSF), a clear liquid surrounding the brain and spinal cord, moves through the brain along a series of channels that surround blood vessels. This system is managed by the glial cells (a brain cell), so the researchers called it the glymphatic system. The glymphatic system clears out and recycles all the brain's toxins.

The scientists reported that the glymphatic system can help remove a toxic protein called beta-amyloid from brain tissue. Beta-amyloid is renowned for accumulating in the brains of patients with Alzheimer's disease.

- **Repairs daily wear and tear:** New research indicates that chronic sleep deprivation can lead to irreversible brain damage. Short sleep may also be linked to shrinking brain volume. Scientists have concluded that the deeper stages of sleep are crucial for repairing the body, including the brain.

- **Makes order from chaos:** As you go about your daily activities, your brain is exposed to thousands of stimuli — auditory, visual, and/or neurosensory. And it can't possibly process all that information as it comes in. A lot of tagging and archiving of memories goes on at night while you are sleeping. People who think they have adapted well to sleeping just four or five hours a night are often wrong; memory tests show they are not functioning optimally.

- **Creates memories:** One of the chemicals involved in creating memories, acetylcholine, is also involved in sleep and dreaming. What happens in people who start to develop Alzheimer's is the brain cells that produce acetylcholine are destroyed, so people stop dreaming as much. Interestingly, a side effect of the most used drug to treat Alzheimer's, Aricept, is its ability to induce vivid dreams.

Four Long-Standing Theories of Sleep

- **Inactivity theory** — sleep keeps us out of harm's way at night-time.
- **Energy Conservation theory** — sleep reduces our energy demand and expenditure.
- **Restorative theory** — sleep provides an opportunity for the body to repair and rejuvenate.
- **Brain Plasticity theory** — sleep is needed for learning, memory, and brain development.

Sleep Disturbances

The health consequences of sleep disturbances are dire:

- **Emotional** - impacts feelings, HPA (hypothalamus, Pituitary, Adrenal Axis) results in overt negative behaviors such as anger, substance abuse, poor motor control
- **Cognitive** - impacts attention, memory, and executive function
- **Physical** - reduces immunity, increases your risk of cancer, cardiovascular disease, diabetes, and metabolic issues
- **Brain Health** - Neurotransmitter Release and Sleep are intimately intertwined. Psychiatric and neurodegenerative diseases are often concurrent with some form of sleep/circadian rhythm disruption

Risks Associated with Sleep Deprivation

- Increased risk of car accidents
- Increased accidents at work
- Reduced ability to learn or remember
- Reduced productivity at work
- Reduced creativity at work or in other activities
- Reduced athletic performance
- Increased risk of Type 2 Diabetes, obesity, cancer, high blood pressure, osteoporosis, and cardiovascular disease
- Increased risk of depression
- Increased risk of dementia and Alzheimer's disease
- Decreased immune function
- Slowed reaction time
- Reduced regulation of emotions and emotional perception
- Poor grades in school
- Increased susceptibility to stomach ulcers
- Exacerbates current chronic diseases such as Alzheimer's, Parkinson's, Multiple Sclerosis
- Cutting one hour of sleep a night increases the expression of genes associated with inflammation, immune excitability, diabetes cancer risk, and stress
- Contributes to premature aging by interfering with growth hormone production, normally released by your pituitary gland during deep sleep

Sleep, Neuroplasticity, and Memory

Your brain is taking in a massive amount of information every day. It is up to the brain to determine what is important, what you learned, and what should be kept in memory. This is a huge job! Thankfully our brain clears most of the information we take in. Either the signal wasn't strong enough (not important), or fuzzy (no clear signal); our brain would be on overload if we remembered absolutely everything. This process of determining what our brain keeps and uses and what it gets rid of happens when we sleep.

When we sleep — and this includes napping — our brain is very busy. I have already mentioned several of the tasks it performs while sleeping. Memory formation and consolidation are some of the most critical functions while we are sleeping. As we gather information while we are awake, it is first contained within short-term memory. As we sleep, this information is moved on to the hippocampus — the center of learning and memory. We have two hippocampi – one on each side of our brain. The hippocampus is very busy during the time we are awake. So, when the inputs are quiet the hippocampus gets busy consolidating memories.

Well, what does that mean?

When the signal of the input is strong enough, the hippocampus scans the brain to determine if there is another memory like it. If there is, the memories are consolidated into a single memory.

What happens then?

The consolidated memories are stronger — meaning that you can recall faster and easier. It also changes that memory a slight bit. Because the memory is consolidated, you don't quite remember it the way it might have happened.

You can experience this: Say you had a group of friends when you were younger, and you all had the same experiences. You would think you would all recall these experiences with the same detail. However, each of you has a lifetime of memory consolidation going on from the individual experiences you have all had. Let's say you have a reunion and start talking about old times. The major theme of the memory would be similar but each of you would have your version of the memory because you have each added your similar memories, and now the group memory is flavored with all your memories that have been consolidated with it.

Preferentially, the hippocampus encodes explicit memories (requires conscious thoughts such as recalling who came to dinner) and those that have behavioral relevance to the individual. There is growing evidence that explicit encoding, even in procedural tasks, involves a dialect between the prefrontal cortex and the hippocampus. Get good sleep and make your memories.

The Neuroscience of Dreams

I am not going to delve into what dreams mean or the specifics of dreaming. This is just a slight reference to the neuroscience of dreams.

Dreams occur in both REM and NREM sleep, but the characteristics differ:

- REM dreams (rapid eye movement) – long, mostly visual, and usually not connected to the immediate events of the day
- NREM dreams (non-rapid eye movement – referred to as deep or slow wave sleep)– shorter, less visual, less emotional, more conceptual, and usually related to the current life of the dreamer

Sleep Apnea

Obstructive sleep apnea is a common and serious sleep disorder that causes you to stop breathing during sleep. In many cases, an apnea, or temporary pause in breathing, is caused by the tissue in the back of the throat collapsing. The muscles of the upper airway relax when you fall asleep. If you sleep on your back, gravity can cause the tongue to fall back. This narrows the airway and reduces the amount of air that can reach your lungs. The narrowed airway causes snoring by making the tissue in the back of the throat vibrate as you breathe. There is some thought that sleep apnea may be an issue of aging. The tissue in the back of the throat is no longer elastic enough and just collapses. Because of that, breathing pauses can last from a few seconds to a few minutes. These pauses may occur 30 or more times per hour.

How does that affect us? We end up suffering from hypoxia, which is a lack of oxygen to the brain and the heart. The results are very damaging. Because the brain and heart don't get the oxygen they need, you are at a greater risk of heart disease and cognitive impairment. Other health issues that arise due to sleep apnea are high blood pressure, stroke, pre-diabetes diabetes, and depression.

Common symptoms of sleep apnea arc:

- Loud or frequent snoring
- Silent pauses in breathing
- Choking or gasping sounds
- Daytime sleepiness or fatigue
- Unrefreshing sleep
- Insomnia
- Morning headaches
- Nocturia
- Difficulty concentrating
- Memory loss
- Irritability

Risk factors:

- Excess weight
- Having a large neck size (17 inches or more)
- Middle age
- Male gender
- Hypertension
- Or a family history of sleep apnea

Tips for Good Sleep Hygiene

- Exercise regularly, but not within a few hours of bedtime.
- Eat a balanced diet, and don't eat heavy meals before bedtime.
- Practice relaxation techniques at bedtime, such as deep breathing, visualization, or meditation.
- Avoid caffeine, nicotine, and alcohol in the afternoon and evening hours.
- Set a regular bedtime and waking hours.
- If you do not fall asleep within 20 minutes of going to bed, get up and do something else until you feel tired.
- Keep a sleep journal to track activities, food, and drink, emotional circumstances, or other factors that might influence how well you sleep.
- Keep a steady room temperature in your bedroom (not too warm).
- Avoid reading, conversing, and watching television in bed.
- Make the bedroom a safe place, with locks on the door, a smoke alarm, a telephone, and good lighting within reach of the bed. [13]

CALM / STRESS

This is the last section of the Healthy Brain for Life Plan! Let's finish this lifestyle plan off with a lesson about stress. This is something that most of us probably experience in our lives. I will talk about the different types of stress and how they impact our bodies and our brains. You will see how some types of stress are good for your brain and how chronic stress can destroy brain cells.

Then I will finish up this lesson with suggestions on how to reset your stress response and build resilience to it.

What Is Stress?

A primary function of our brain is to help us survive. When our brain is threatened, it goes into the fight or flight response well before we are even aware of the threat. This response is critical to our survival. Stress is the highly orchestrated response to a real or imagined threat or challenge. Note the word "imagined" here. This response includes body, mind, emotions, and thought processes. Even though this system was necessary for our prehistoric ancestors to keep them alive, we live in a different environment now. The prolonged effect of stress has a toxic effect on our brains and our body. The response that kept our primitive ancestors alive is now killing us.

There are two biological stress pathways. Again – pay attention to the word "biological."

The Neurosymphony of Stress

It is not necessary to remember the parts of the brain involved in the stress response. I have presented them to you so that you understand the complexity of the Autonomic Nervous System. It is the nitty-gritty of the stress response. Just read it and breathe!

- **The Autonomic Nervous System**: the part of the nervous system responsible for the control of bodily functions not consciously directed, such as breathing, the heartbeat, and the digestive system.

How does your brain know that you are threatened? When faced with stressors, the brain's "extended amygdala" processes fear, threats, and anxiety and encodes emotional states. The extended amygdala is composed of the amygdala and the nucleus accumbens. Extended amygdala neurons send axons or connections to the hypothalamus and other midbrain structures that are involved in the expression of emotional responses.

The autonomic nervous system is the rapid response system for stress/threat. Two systems in the autonomic nervous system are responsible for the first reaction to stress:

- **Sympathetic Nervous System** – this turns on the fight or flight response. SNS activates the adrenal medulla (which is on the kidneys) and releases adrenalin and norepinephrine. This is the fight-or-flight response.
- **Parasympathetic Nervous System** – promotes the relaxation response. It uses acetylcholine to get to the rest and digest phase.

- The trouble is that some stress hormones don't know when to quit. They remain active in the brain for too long, injuring and even killing cells in the hippocampus, which is the area of your brain needed for learning and memory. Because of the hierarchal dominance of the SNS over the PNS, it often requires conscious effort to initiate your relaxation response and reestablish metabolic equilibrium.
- **HPA Axis and cortisol slow response**
- The **hypothalamus** integrates bodily functions for the maintenance of homeostasis (balance of body systems). It is extensively connected with the autonomic nervous system, the **neuroendocrine system** (made up of nerves and gland cells that make hormones and release them into the bloodstream), and the **limbic system** (part of the brain involved in our behavioral and emotional responses).
- The stress response acting via the HPA axis results in adrenal glands releasing cortisol, which induces metabolic effects. Cortisol also acts on the hypothalamus and pituitary gland by negative feedback.
- **Cortisol** is the "Goldilocks hormone" because you must have just the right amount to be healthy.

Stress Effects on the Body

First, your body is primed for survival. In the acute stage of stress, after all the hormones have been released, your senses become more acute; your memory is sharpened; and you feel less sensitive to pain. When you are on alert, you have increased strength, endurance, and energy. This allows for your fight-or-flight response. You are primed for survival.

Stress Effects on the Brain

In this acute stage, the neurochemical, norepinephrine, is released. This chemical neurotransmitter creates new memories, improves mood, encourages creative thinking, and stimulates the brain to increase cognitive reserve (new connections in the brain).

Short-term stress is an asset and can allow great things to happen. Our challenge becomes using this short-term stress as a tool and not letting it escalate and stick around to become chronic stress.

What Does Stress Do to the Brain?

As a reminder, there are two types of stress:

Acute stress enhances attention and memory formation. Without this, you would never learn new things, get motivated, or achieve your goals or your deadlines.

The **chronic stress** cycle has cortisol staying way too long in your brain. Even though it initially puts you into fight-or-flight mode and helps your brain be more effective, on a long-term basis it can kill brain cells. This is not a good thing.

Researchers from the Yale Stress Center found that chronic stress can reduce brain volume, which is where cells are dying, and a decrease in brain function in otherwise healthy individuals. They found that stress can hurt you now by decreasing the amount of gray matter, but it can also make it more difficult to manage stress in the future. The continual release of stress hormones adversely affects brain function, particularly memory.

Chronic stress changes your brain chemistry, can create traumatic memories, develop mood and anxiety disorders, and increase the risk of dementia. Too much stress prevents the birth of new brain cells as well as impacts the connections between brain cells (which are made up of cognitive reserve).

The Effects of Chronic Stress on Your Body

Chronic stress has its signature on our bodies. You even experience physical changes in this state.

- The endocrine system – we are constantly triggering the endocrine system, which is responsible for growth and development.
- Homeostasis (internal balance) – our body is a very fine-tuned being and everything works together. Homeostasis or balance makes sure that no system is out of whack.
- Metabolism – these are body energy levels.
- Reproduction – if you suffer from chronic stress, it may affect your fertility.
- Response to stimuli – stress and/or injury.
- In the chronic stress state, you can gain weight and have increased blood sugar due to the pancreas malfunctioning.

7. The pancreas gets overwhelmed with the increased amounts of blood sugar it needs to process.
8. Your blood pressure is elevated, and you deposit fats into your blood.
9. This puts your cardiovascular system at great risk for heart attacks and strokes.

The Effects of Chronic Stress on Your Brain

Now let's look at our brain under siege from chronic stress.

1. Stress affects your whole body, and it dramatically changes and impacts your brain.

2. Two areas of the brain are specifically affected.

- Hippocampus: the center for new learning and memory.

- Amygdala: the emotional control center of our brain.

Researchers at UC Berkley found that chronic stress, through the actions of the stress hormone cortisol, causes the brain to hardwire connections between the hippocampus and the amygdala, creating a vicious cycle of fight-or-flight response.

- Chronic stress causes brain cells to inhibit connections to the prefrontal cortex, where learning, memory, and executive function occur and sets the brain up for depression and anxiety.
- Research also indicated that chronic stress causes a decrease in brain cells that mature into neurons while affecting learning and memory capabilities.

The Power of Cortisol

The Dana Institute of Brain Research published that cortisol is so powerful that it can:

- alter the structure of neurons,
- affect their connections,
- influence behavior, and
- change hormonal processes.

This results in increased anxiety, decreased memory, and decreased cognitive function.

Cortisol kills brain cells.

Studies have shown that cortisol can damage and kill cells in the hippocampus. There is evidence that chronic stress can cause premature brain aging. Yale researchers found that stress reduces brain volume and function in otherwise healthy individuals. Finally, cortisol has been shown to make your brain more vulnerable to strokes, aging, and stressful events. Cortisol also hinders the function of neurotransmitters – the chemicals the brain cells use to communicate with each other. Excessive cortisol makes it difficult to think and retrieve long-term memories. In a crisis, people can get confused because their mind goes blank due to excess cortisol. These memories can be just general knowledge like how to get out of a building as an example.

Building Resilience to Stress

It is possible to build resilience to stress. You can do this through rewarding social experiences. These are associated with the release of inner opioids and oxytocin (which is the connecting, bonding hormone) and the neuromodulator dopamine (which is the reward, motivating neurochemical) – that may protect against elevated glucocorticoids (a kind of steroid). Cortisol is the most important of the glucocorticoid or steroid hormone group.

The effects of stress vary at different stages of life with early childhood, adolescence, and aging — the most vulnerable periods.

Building resilience is about how well your brain handles stress and involves staying or getting back to the window of tolerance in a zone when the nervous system is relaxed, calm, alert, and engaged. Resilience is:

- Getting the prefrontal cortex back online by learning to recognize triggers that set off a stress response when you are not in danger.
- Engaging socially – reach out to friends and family; social connections buffer stress.
- Cultivating optimism – seek out and savor positive emotions.
- Exercising daily and sleeping nightly.
- Doing something new – novel and challenging experiences inoculate you against future stress.
- Engaging in mindful meditation:

- Mindfulness intentionally brings our attention back to the senses.
- Doing this repeatedly activates the prefrontal cortex regions associated with being present, and those areas grow stronger.
- We rewire our brains to be present – and be healthier and happier.

Worry and Anxiety Feed the Chronic Stress Cycle

How to Stop Worrying: Self-Help Strategies for Anxiety Relief

Self-Help Tip #1: Create a worry period

1. Trying to stop anxious thoughts doesn't work; try to distract, ignore, or suppress your worrying thoughts for as long as you can — only to find them bouncing back stronger than ever. Stopping thoughts brings attention to the very thoughts you are trying to ignore. Because they have taken prominence in your mind, these thoughts seem even more important now.
2. Learning to postpone worrying:

- **Create a worry period**: Choose a time and a place for worrying. It should be the same time every day and early enough that it won't make you anxious before you go to bed. You can worry about everything during this time. The rest of the day is off-limits to these problems.
- **Postpone your worry**: If your worry pops into your head during the day, make a note of it and worry about it during your designated worry time. Reassure yourself that you will be thinking about this later and then go on with your day. Repeat if necessary.

- **Go over your worry list during the worry period.** Review and reflect on your list. If you have thoughts about your worries, indulge those but only for the allotted time. If your worry has resolved before your worry time, let it go cut your worry period down, and enjoy the rest of the day.

Self-help tip #2: Ask yourself if the problem is solvable

Research shows that when you are worrying, you temporarily feel less anxious. Continually running the problem over and over keeps you distracted from your emotions. It deludes you into thinking you are coming up with solutions. The problem with this is that you don't distinguish worrying from actual problem-solving. Problem-solving comes up with actionable steps. Worrying does nothing to come up with a resolution.

- **Distinguish between solvable and unsolvable worries**
  1. Is the problem something that you are currently facing, rather than a what-if?
  2. If the problem is an imaginary what-if, how likely is it to happen? Is your concern realistic?
  3. Can you do something about the problem or prepare for it, or is it out of your control?

Productive, solvable worries are those you can act on immediately. Unproductive worries have no corresponding action. If your problem is solvable, act, and start brainstorming. Make a list of everything you can think of. Focus on the things you have the power to change. Plan actions after reviewing your options. You will stop worrying when you feel like you are doing something about the problem.

- **Dealing with unsolvable worries**

If you are a chronic worrier, most of your problems will fall into this category. When that is the case, you need to tune into your emotions. Worrying helps you avoid unpleasant emotions. While you are worrying, your emotions are suppressed. As soon as you stop, the tension and anxiety come storming back. It is necessary to embrace your feelings if you want to break this cycle. You must come to an understanding that your emotions can be messy and scary. But, when you accept that your emotions are what make you human; you can experience them without becoming overwhelmed and learn how to use them to your advantage.

Self-help tip #3: Accept uncertainty

Chronic worriers cannot stand unpredictability and doubt. They need to know without any uncertainty what's going to happen. To them, worrying is a way to predict the future, prevent unpleasant surprises, and control the outcome. But this doesn't work! Thinking about everything that could go wrong doesn't make life predictable. It is just an illusion to believe that you are safer. Focusing on worst-case scenarios won't keep those things from happening. If you want to get past this block, you need to start addressing your need for certainty and immediate answers.

Self-help tip #4: Challenge anxious thoughts

Here is a real conundrum: If you are a worrier and have anxiety, you probably look at the world in ways that make it far more dangerous than it is. For example, you may overestimate the possibility that things will turn out badly, jump to immediate worst-case scenarios, or treat every negative thought as if it were a fact. You may believe that you are incapable of taking care of life's problems and just fall apart. This is known as cognitive distortion. These thoughts are not based on reality, but they can be very difficult to give up. They are so automatic because they are on a subconscious level, and you are not even aware that you are thinking this way. To break this thinking you must retrain your brain.

Self-help tip #5: Be aware of how others affect you

How you feel is affected by the company you keep. Research has shown that emotions are contagious. We are affected by moods from everyone — even strangers. The people you spend the most time with affect you the most.

- Spend less time with people who make you anxious. If there are people in your life who constantly make you feel bad, spend less time with them or establish new relationship boundaries.
- Choose your confidantes wisely. When you are anxious, know who you can talk to. Some people will help you gain perspective while others will feed into your fears and worries.
- Let your worries go. When you don't try to control your anxious thoughts, they will pass. Only when you engage in your worries will you get stuck.

- Stay focused on the present. Pay attention to how your body feels, the rhythm of your breathing, your ever-changing emotions, and the thoughts that cross your mind. Continue to bring your thoughts back to the present.

Self-help tip #6: Practice mindfulness

Worrying is usually focused on the future. Mindfulness will help bring you back to the present. This practice is based on acknowledging the thought and then letting it go.

- Acknowledge and observe your anxious thoughts and feelings. Don't follow your old patterns of fighting or avoiding your thoughts. Observe them with no reaction or judgment.

Mindfulness

Mindfulness is wonderful and initially difficult. I learned mindfulness several years ago, and it made a significant difference in my life. Then my time became scarcer for practice, and I gradually stopped. Then life took a chunk of me, so I decided that I had to make the time to practice mindfulness again. Chronic stress worries and anxieties take a toll on your body, brain, and life. We do have control over all of this. One of the mantras I constantly tell myself is: "Change your thoughts and change your life." It is worth the effort. [18]

Adapted from: How to Stop Worrying – Self-Help Strategies for Anxiety Relief. Retrieved from http://www.helpguide.org/articles/how-to-stop-worrying.htm

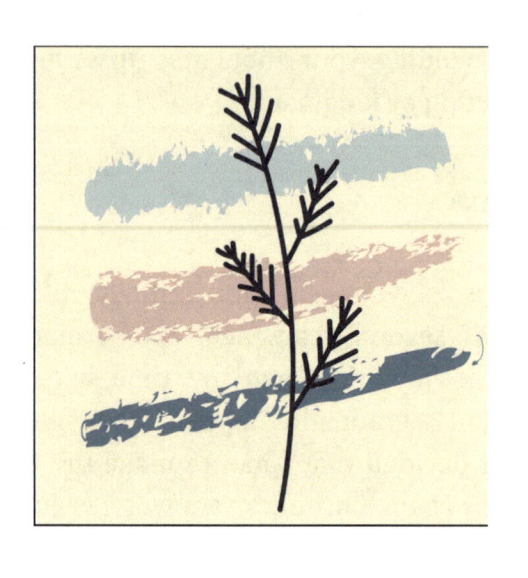

chapter nine

The Keys to Successful Longevity

Longevity sounds fantastic. But if you are sick and suffer from cognitive decline, it is a nightmare. All the information you just read through might have left you overwhelmed. Let's unwrap all the pieces to the puzzle. It is time to create your journey through healthy aging.

An aging body has an impact on an aging brain. Your overall physical health is critical to brain health. Take a complete look at your health and health issues. Are you taking care of yourself? Successful aging requires that you put yourself first. Are you doing everything possible to live a healthy life? That is where your first focus of action should be. Get a physical, be current with your vaccinations, be current with your dental and vision appointments, and get your hearing checked. You see your body every day and you can see what is going on with your health. There is no second-guessing about what is happening.

Now, let's look at the aging brain. Your physical health impacts how fast your brain is aging because our brain does not know how old you are. Your brain ages by the lifestyle you lead!

Whereas we can see physical aging, we are at a loss about our brain age. Just look at it this way — If you are healthy and your brain is firing on all cylinders, your brain might be younger than your chronological age. This is what we aim for, and this is why you just read all the inside stories of your aging brain.

It was necessary to discuss normal brain aging changes. My experience in speaking with older adults is that they are often fearful that they are experiencing the beginnings of dementia. Understanding that these brain changes are part of the aging process does relieve many people's fears. However, it is important to understand that age is a nonmodifiable risk factor for dementia. The older you get your risk of getting Alzheimer's increases.

That took us to the magic of neuroplasticity and neurogenesis. Our ability to create new neurons and synaptic connections is our means of changing our brains.

Of course, the way we live our lives has an impact on losses our brains sustain. Most of us are entering our older years with a chronic health condition, or we have held on to habits that have impaired our physical health. Your chronic disease is with you forever. You must take care of yourself to keep your chronic disease under control. When you do that, you reduce the risk factors for developing dementia.

Calculate your total risk factors (Chapter Seven). That is

your baseline. If you have diabetes, heart disease, kidney disease, or any other chronic condition under control, you can decrease that risk factor.

The non-modifiable risk factors cannot be changed. Your age, gender, and genetic factors that belong to you — are yours. These risk factors must be considered when you put together your lifestyle plan.

Lifestyle is responsible for 70% of developing dementia. How high is your risk factor number? The good news is, you have the power to change that number by the lifestyle that you lead. That takes you to your lifestyle plan.

How to incorporate lifestyle changes into your life without upending your life.

First, check into your lifestyle as it is right now. Maybe you are already leading a brain-healthy lifestyle.

- Do you sit most of the day or are you up moving around?
- Are you bored and listless?
- Is processed food your dinner of choice?
- Over the years, have you isolated yourself from friends or family?
- Do you feel that your life has meaning and purpose?
- What about sleep? Do you feel rested when you wake?
- Have you learned to navigate the stress cycle?

These are just some random questions about lifestyle. Be honest with yourself when you start to think about your answers. There is no right or wrong answer but honesty about your lifestyle is imperative.

MOVE / Physical Exercise

Remember that all parts of the brain-healthy lifestyle are important. Review what you are already doing to stay healthy. If you already exercise, look closely at what type of exercise you are doing. You need to get your heart beating a little faster to get the blood, carbs, and oxygen to your brain for energy and to stimulate new neuronal growth.

Here are some ideas to get you started:

- Take daily or nightly walks with family or friends.
- Physical exercise two or three times per week reduces the risk of Alzheimer's.
- Pickleball is sweeping the nation for participants of all ages. It is a perfect exercise to get your heart beating, hone spatial-relationship skills, and challenge your balance.
- Get a pedometer or use your smartphone to keep track of your steps per day. Aim high —7,500 steps per day!
- Consider dance classes. Pattern dance, waltz, tango, or polka all work great. If you are ambitious, try out those jitterbug steps from long ago.
- If you can't do aerobic exercises that involve walking or dancing, try some of the chair yoga classes, or yoga

for seniors. These exercises are not only good for your heart, but they are good for flexibility.

- Swimming provides no impact aerobic exercise. Find water exercise classes to get that low-impact aerobics benefit.
- Put some resistance training in your exercise schedule. Resistance training improves muscle mass and increases metabolism.
- Keep a journal of the benefits you experience from exercising.

As I move through each of the pieces of the brain-healthy lifestyle, I want you to keep in mind that you need to incorporate these practices into your life. It is too difficult to center your life around these changes. You need to fit these practices into your life. Take these suggestions on physical exercise and implement them into practices you are already doing. It must become a habit — something that you don't have to think about to do it.

Challenge / Mental Stimulation

Challenging your brain might feel more difficult. But I bet you are already putting your brain to the test every day. It doesn't have to be something formal, like studying a language or learning an instrument. Planting a new garden is stimulating or learning some new dance steps. Check out what is going on around you wherever you live. You need to get your new brain cells to work, or your brain will prune them out. You can't change your brain if you don't stimulate it. Can't think of anything to do right now? Check these suggestions and see if a couple of ideas fit.

Here are some ideas to get you started:

- Participate in activities that are creative and artistic.
- Establish a night a week for family board games, card games, or interactive games. Get everyone involved.
- Go to museums, plays, and even neighborhood amateur productions. Discuss whatever you saw, learned, or participated in.
- Learn a second language.
- Join a book club — read and discuss books of all kinds.
- Travel – it can even be to a different part of town where you are not familiar with the route to get there, shops and restaurants that are new to you.
- Volunteer.
- Enjoy the music – from playing an instrument to listening to a concert.
- Enroll in online brain training. Stick with it and see if it makes a difference in your brain function.

Nourish / Nutrition

As the research for a healthy brain continues, nutrition is coming up big! Our entire body and brain need nutritional support. This can be a little more daunting if you have eaten the same foods all your life, and if those foods don't support your health. Remember though, this is not a diet. This is a day-in and day-out way to stay healthy and keep your brain young. The section on nutrition is very complete but here are a few suggestions for you to start integrating good foods into your life.

Here are some ideas to get you started:

- Take a list of brain-healthy foods and make a trip to the grocery store. Consciously try to buy foods that will support your brain-healthy lifestyle and make your recipes more brain-healthy.

- Keep a basket of fresh fruits that are filled with brain-boosting antioxidants in your kitchen.

- Consider keeping a journal for two weeks of what you eat daily. This can help you become conscious of what you are eating and perhaps why you eat certain foods. You might be surprised how much easier it is to incorporate more brain-healthy foods into your diet.

- Finally, if you find this too difficult to put together, remember to fill your plate with primarily green vegetables, and dark-skinned fruit, and keep your meat intake to once or twice a week. Eat Smart and eat Clean. Whole foods without additives will improve your health.

Connect / Socialization

Now we need to get out into the world and be with other people. As it was mentioned, we are hardwired to connect. It is critical for building cognitive reserve. If you have family and friends, call them, and start setting aside time to see them. The key here is "see." We need to have our group, our tribe, our friends. If you have kept to yourself for a while, gently ease yourself into discovering new places where you can meet like-minded people.

Here are some ideas to get you started:

- Invite friends and family to your home.
- Have fun together. Play board games, complete a jigsaw puzzle, or just talk.
- Make plans with friends and family to do something new — like going to a museum, seeing a play, or going to a sporting event.
- Find out if there are any book clubs or discussion groups you can join.
- See what your local community center has to offer.
- Seek out lecture series within the community that you can attend (e.g., OLLI – Osher Lifelong Learning Institute – usually in partnership with local universities).
- Volunteer, mentor, and become active in a charity or other community organization.
- Use modern technology to increase socialization. Become part of the social network.

Sleep

Did you ever think that sleep is so important to brain health? We are amazing creations. Sleep not only refreshes our body, but it cleans our brains and embeds our memories of the day. Incredible! But if you can't sleep, your physical and brain functioning take a nosedive. Look over these suggestions for getting a night's worth of restful sleep.

Here are some ideas to get you started:

- Keep a sleep journal to track:
- Your bedtime routine and note any of the activities that might interfere with sleep.
- Your sleep patterns and see how close you're waking and sleeping times coincide with normal circadian rhythms.
- If you are having memory problems, look at your sleeping habits and routines. Note if you are taking sleeping medications. Sleeping medications are not meant for long-term use.
- Work towards achieving healthy sleep patterns including an awareness of how easily you can "talk" yourself into insomnia.
- Find out if you snore during the night. Check with your doctor about having a sleep study done to determine the cause of your snoring.
- Keep a journal by your bed and write down your dreams when you wake up.

Calm / Stress

The section on stress is long because stress is so ingrained in our lives, we need to understand how it is impacting us.

When you are doing your lifestyle review, pay attention to how stress has affected your life. We consider it just part of our everyday life, but we don't pay attention to what it is doing to us – in the moment and throughout our lifetime. How do you break the stress cycle? Here are some suggestions for getting you started to bounce back from stress.

Here are some ideas to get you started:

- Keep a stress journal — see if you can figure out the trigger for your stress.
- Record how you react to stressful events.
- Practice taking a deep breath to quiet your reactions when you are in the middle of a stressful event.
- Practice written responses to use when diffusing stress.
- Have a planned reaction to stress — take a walk, do yoga, pray, meditate – whatever you need to get you centered.
- Practice being optimistic — even in the face of stress.
- Surround yourself with family and friends — know who has your back in tough situations.

My hope in writing this book was to educate you on what is happening to you and how it affects your older years. It is never too late to start a brain-healthy lifestyle and you are never too old to change your brain.

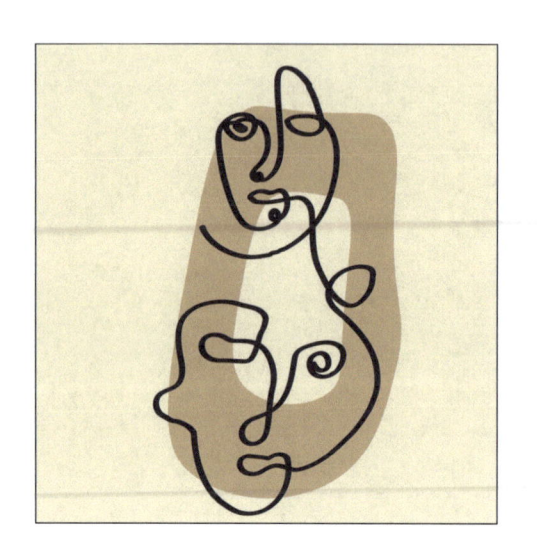

chapter ten

Meet My Mom

Over the years I have studied the brain, brain health and the brain-healthy lifestyle. What I discovered was that learning the science was the easy part of this new field. Applying that knowledge to everyday life was more complicated. In this book I introduced ways to incorporate the lifestyle into your life, without upending your life. Because this lifestyle knowledge might be new to you, it is still necessary to focus on each new step you take to make this change a normal way of life. Even though your brain loves this challenge, it still might feel overwhelming at the beginning of this experience. There is so much angst over changing the lifestyle you have lived for most of your life that people give up before they even try. "It's too hard," is what I hear the most. However, you may be living more of this lifestyle than you ever imagined. To give you a real example of this, I want to introduce my mom.

My mom was 91years old when she died. That day she met with her friends, Geri and Carol, and they had lunch and played cards. Talking to them afterward, we learned that they had a great time talking, laughing, and socializing over their card games. These three friends checked on each other every day during Covid lockdown. Their friendship was deep. Mom then stopped at the store and bought a few groceries, but as soon as she walked through the door of her apartment she collapsed and died! We found out later that she had a heart attack. What a wonderful way to go!

She didn't focus on a brain-healthy life. She didn't even know what that meant until she came to my presentations and learned all about it. But she did live a brain-healthy lifestyle.

When mom was growing up there was no fast food, no TV, and neighborhoods were tight. Everyone grew up together. My grandmother was an excellent cook and baker. Her days of the week were divided into baking days, laundry days, and every day was about keeping up with 14 children. The years of childbearing were long. So, the oldest helped take care of the youngest and the family unit supported each other. And there was another bond that kept the family together — their Catholic faith. My mom was steadfast in her faith, and I would even say that is what supported her through the toughest parts of her life. This foundation of support through family and faith would serve mom well throughout her entire life.

I remember stories of mom when she was a teenager. There were many happy stories about dances that she went to with her friends and sisters. Mom loved to dance. She and dad would act silly and would dance around our tiny house. There was a lot of laughter throughout my youth. It was the tradition at that time that the dad would go to work and the mom would stay home and take care of the house and kids. That was the way we lived; but with so many kids and only one bread earner, money was tight. Mom cooked everything from scratch, there was no fast food then or processed food to have a quick meal. It was a treat to go to Burger King. We were excited when Chef Boyardee had a pizza mix. It helped that we had never really eaten good pizza before so what tasted like cardboard with tomato sauce and a little parmesan cheese was fantastic.

This sounds idyllic and for us, maybe it was. Even though mom could squeeze a dollar out of a quarter, dad was always looking for a second job. Being from a big family we had many cousins older than us. It was always exciting when a box of "slightly used" clothes showed up at our door. Dad and mom would convince us that "these clothes were as good as new." For us, they were new. The extended family always had our back.

Then the unthinkable happened. My dad went into the hospital with seizures when I was 17 and a senior in high school. Once he went into the hospital, he never came back out. Dad was 44 when he died, and mom had just turned 40 the week before his death. She now had six kids at home, ages 2 – 17. All our lives were changed forever.

I got married two years after dad's death, so I really didn't see the impact of mom being a widow had on the younger kids. It was years later when my younger sisters and brother told me about the lengths mom went to in creating such a fulfilling life for each of them. She was the most resilient person I have ever known. As I learned throughout my studies, resilience is a learned skill and critical to a healthy brain lifestyle.

The friendships you had as a married person completely change when you are widowed. She hated feeling like a fifth wheel and started pulling back from those friends. Amazingly, she was able to stay home from working until my youngest sister was five and in kindergarten. Mom went out and found a job for the first time in twenty years! And this was the first time that she started making new friends.

Being connected to others was part of my mom's DNA. Throughout her life, as family and friends started to die, she would find new friends to be with. She never wallowed in her circumstances. I became the designated partner taking her to funerals. It was so tough, but mom was tough. Mom lived in a high-rise apartment in the same area where she grew up. She went to the same church (St. Boniface) all her life. One afternoon she was at Mass, and she noticed one of her friends who ran in the same high school crowd that she was in. He had lost his wife a while ago and when he saw mom, he asked her if she wanted to have an early dinner. They talked and laughed about old times and old friends. (I was so happy when she was telling me about this!). He asked her if she would like to go out again sometime and she readily agreed. Because he didn't know where she lived, she asked him to follow her to her apartment and stop up and have a drink! Mom is telling me this story very calmly and I was happy to hear that she might have a companion to go out with. Then she tells me that she was fixing his drink and when she turned around, HE WAS DEAD!! I was speechless but I finally asked what she did next. She stayed composed and called 911 and they transported his body to the morgue. But it was up to her to call his kids and tell them what happened.

Apparently she wasn't mortified to tell them that their dad died in her apartment. Their response was that they were glad he died with her (they knew her). Thank goodness mom had a great sense of humor because her sons-in-law teased her incessantly about having a dead man in her apartment!

Once mom started working, she never looked back. Her last job was at the YWCA of Greater Cincinnati. It turned out to be the perfect job for her. She retired at age 65 and then the next week she went back to work for the "Y" on a part-time basis. The "Y" paid their employees once a month and mom worked on payroll the week before checks were issued. In that role she had to go to several classes for different computer programs for payroll. No doubt she was the oldest person in the class and even though it took her a little longer to feel comfortable, she did it! Shortly after she turned 85, she was informed that they were going to upgrade programs again. This time she retired — for real!

The YWCA was in downtown Cincinnati and mom chose to ride the bus. The week she worked she got lots of exercise walking. It served her well. She had a couple of chronic diseases, but her active lifestyle kept them under control.

There are some criteria common to super agers that applied to mom. I don't believe she was a super ager, but she had these attributes.

1. Her faith sustained her through the best and worse times of her life. She was my prayer warrior.
2. There was a lot of stress for mom throughout her life. But she was resilient. Resilience is critical to navigate through tragedies and come back cognitively stronger than ever. Mom had her share of those.
3. Fast food and ultra-processed food where not part of mom's life when she was young, and they were too expensive for a large family when she was older. Whole foods were part of her life and part of ours.
4. She didn't think of herself as physically active, but she was always moving. Walking to the bus and back home and walking through downtown kept her healthy in her later years.
5. Mom always had friends. When friends and family died, she would meet new friends. She was a social person and being connected to others builds cognitive reserve. I believe that was critical to her being cognitively intact when she died.

This was my mom's life which happened to be a brain-healthy life. She didn't worry or stress about getting older. She adapted and changed organically to the circumstances of the life she led.

sources

Chapter Three:

1. Nichols, H. (September 9, 2020. What happens to the brain as we age? https://www.medicalnewstoday.com/articles/319185#Therapies-to-help-slowbrain-aging 2. Heather Walker. (March 01, 2014). *Scientific American MIND.*

Chapter Four:

3. Merzenich, M. (April 2006). Growing evidence of brain plasticity. https://ted.com/talks/Michael_merzenich_growing_evidence_of_brain_plasticity?language=en

Chapter Six:

4. 7UT Health, San Antonio. Glenn Briggs Institute for Alzheimer's and Neurodegenerative Diseases. https://biggsinstitute.org

5. Sandoiu, A. (January 25, 2121). Covid-19 and the brain. What do we know so far? https://www.medicalnewstoday.com/articles/how-does-sars-cov-2-affect-the-brain#Once-it-infects-the-brain-it-can-affect-anything

6. Stevens, R. How does coronavirus affect the brain? https://www.hopkinsmedicine.org/health/conditions-anddiseases/coronavirus/how-does-coronavirus-affect-the-brain

Chapter Seven:

7. WebMD. Medically reviewed by Carol Sarlissian, MD. (May 27, 2022). Things that raise your chances of dementia.

8. Alzheimer's Society. (June 2021). Risk factors for dementia. https://www.alzheimers.org.uk

9. Alzheimer's Society. High blood pressure and dementia. https://www.alzheimer's.org.uk/about-dementia/risk-factors-and-prevention/high-blood-pressure

10. (John Hopkins Bloomberg School of Public Health. (November 12, 2021). Hearing loss and the dementia connection. https://publichealth.jhu.edu/2012/hearingloss-and-the-dementia-connection)

11. Bakalar, N. (June 22, 2015). Pollution may age the brain. The New York Times. http://well.blogs.nytimes.com/2015/06/22/pollution-may-age-the-brain/

12. Queensland Brain Institute. Dementia risk factors. https://qbi.uq.edu.au/dementia/dementia-risk-factors

Chapter Eight:

13. Staying Sharp: Memory and Aging NRTA (AARP's Education Community and the Dana Alliance for BrainInitiatives

14. American Psychological Association. (2008). Understanding aging brains, how to improve memory, and when to seek help. https://www.apa.org/aging-older-adults/memory-brain-changes

15. Wadyka, S. (May 4, 2023). Do you know how to spot foods that are ultra-pro-cessed? https://nytimes.com/interactive/2023/05/04/well/eat/ultraprocessedfoods.html

16. Rosen, M. (January 11, 2012). Live the life you love! http://www.aarp.org/personal-growth/transitions/info-06-2011/5-weeks-ep5-purpose.html

17. Fredrickson, B. (October 9, 2018). Becoming resilient: an excerpt from Barbara Fredrickson's love 2.0 – creating happiness and health in moments of connection. https://cvdl.ben.edu/blog/becoming-resilient/

18. Azab, M. (January 1, 2021). Meaning and purpose in life (not goals) protect the brain. https://psychologytoday.com/us/blog/neuroscience-in-everyday-life/202101/meaning-and-purpose-in-life-not-goals-protect-the-brain

conclusion

Throughout the 1990s I worked with Physical and Occupational therapists in the long-term care setting. Their primary residents were diagnosed with dementia and lived in the "lock-down" units. I was so upset by what I saw that I was determined to somehow find a better way for these residents to live their final years.

In one week, I registered at the Ohio Academy of Holistic Health to earn a certificate in Clinical Aromatherapy. I knew enough about essential oils to believe that aromatherapy would be a gentle, effective way to ease the difficult behaviors that many people with end-stage Alzheimer's experience. It turned out that I was right.

That same week I registered at Mount St. Joseph University in Cincinnati to earn a BA in Gerontology. Along the way, I received a Nursing Home Administrator's license. As if that wasn't enough, I entered the graduate program at Miami University in Oxford Ohio, and received a Master's in Gerontological Studies degree. My focus throughout this journey was the different aspects of dementia and what I could do to alleviate the suffering of that disease.

The possibilities of making a difference seemed endless while I was in school. The outside world was a whole different ballgame. Clinical aromatherapy was an unknown entity and fear of drifting from traditional procedures caused most facilities to ignore the benefits. I had the nursing home administrator license, so I understood the requirements of care that nursing homes need to adhere to. However, I didn't find my first adopter to trial aromatherapy for the behaviors of dementia. I had to find another pathway to make a difference around dementia.

Learning about the aging brain and the discoveries in brain health was exhilarating! The first articles and research papers that I read made me feel like I had found the fountain of youth. I was experiencing brain aging changes and after seeing firsthand the ravages dementia caused, I was worried. This news was an answer to my prayers. The more I learned, the more excited I got about the possibility of a future without Alzheimer's. It was far too early to see the reality of that, but this new research provided hope.

Again, I was too early with this knowledge to get anyone to listen to me. It was frustrating but I continued to learn more about brain health. These were the years that the leading-edge boomers were in their fifties. Even this early brain health information would have made a difference in the lifestyles boomers lived. They could have decreased their risk factors for dementia.

Now, twenty years later, the leading-edge boomers are well into their seventies. The brain is now taking center stage in health and wellness. The optimum age for this information is the forties and fifties and brain health programs are directed toward this group. That is great news for those in that age group! My feeling is that the boomers believe it is too late for them. Brain aging changes seem to accelerate the older you get. It is scary. The incidence of me knowing someone near my age has Alzheimer's, is devastating. The Boomer Brain was written to educate boomers that it is NEVER too late to change your brain. The evolution of brain science has given way to hope that we can maintain a high-functioning brain until the day we die. This book briefly explains the basic science that has made this statement a reality. My example of coming back from brain surgery and Debbie Hampton's extraordinary experience of recovering from a traumatic brain injury show how powerful our brains are when we know what to do.

The Lifestyle Plan covers the six elements of brain health. It should be noted that each element has a specific job. No one element is more important than another. The synergy of living all these pieces is greater than the sum of the parts. Each part is boosted in effectiveness through the action of all the other parts of the lifestyle. This lifestyle plan is so powerful that the statement 'Alzheimer's can be prevented' was accepted by the International Alzheimer's Association.

Finally, I wanted to make the point that this lifestyle can be implemented within each person's life. No doubt that everyone has some part of this lifestyle that they are already living. We need to take stock of what we are already doing and what we need to implement. This lifestyle was never meant to be overwhelming. When you determine what you need to do, be disciplined with doing it.

about the author

Patricia McCarthy Faust, MGS

Patricia Faust is a gerontologist, specializing in brain aging and brain health. She was born in Cincinnati, Ohio, and has lived her entire life in the Midwest. However, her articles and blogs on brain aging, and brain health have found a global audience. As a Senior Executive Contributor and CREA Global Award winner for Brainz magazine, Patricia's articles are available to a monthly audience of over one million readers. Her blog site, My Boomer Brain, has international readers in Australia, New Zealand, Canada, Europe, and Asia. Selected blog articles are republished quarterly in InFlow magazine, a digital publication out of New Zealand, with subscribers in the U.S., South Africa, and New Zealand. The Boomer Brain speaks to the Boomer concerns of aging, brain health, and dementia, and offers tools and strategies to maintain an ageless brain.

https://myboomerbrain.com

https://twitter.com/pcfaust

https://www.facebook.com/patricia.faust.18

https://linkedin.com/in/patricia-faust-4358037

Made in United States
Troutdale, OR
06/21/2024